The *Essential Clinical Skills for Nurses* series focuses on key clinical skills for nurses and other health professionals. These concise, accessible books assume no prior knowledge and focus on core clinical skills, clearly presenting common clinical procedures and their rationale, together with the essential background theory. Their user-friendly format makes them an indispensable guide to clinical practice for all nurses, especially to student nurses and newly qualified staff.

Other titles in the *Essential Clinical Skills for Nurses* series:

Trauma Care

Initial assessment and management in the emergency department

Edited by
Elaine Cole MSc, BSc,
Pg Dip (ed), RGN

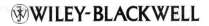

A John Wiley & Sons, Ltd. Publication

This edition first published 2009
© 2009 Blackwell Publishing Ltd

Blackwell Publishing was acquired by John Wiley & Sons in February 2007.
Blackwell's publishing programme has been merged with Wiley's global
Scientific, Technical, and Medical business to form Wiley-Blackwell.

Registered office
John Wiley & Sons Ltd, The Atrium, Southern Gate, Chichester, West Sussex,
PO19 8SQ, United Kingdom

Editorial office
9600 Garsington Road, Oxford, OX4 2DQ, United Kingdom

For details of our global editorial offices, for customer services and for
information about how to apply for permission to reuse the copyright
material in this book please see our website at
www.wiley.com/wiley-blackwell.

Library of Congress Cataloging-in-Publication Data

Trauma care : initial assessment and management in the emergency
department / edited by Elaine Cole.
    p. ; cm. – (Essential clinical skills for nurses)
    Includes bibliographical references and index.
    ISBN 978-1-4051-6230-2 (pbk. : alk. paper)   1. Wounds and
injuries–Nursing.   2. Emergency nursing.   I. Cole, Elaine.   II. Series.
    [DNLM: 1. Wounds and Injuries–diagnosis.   2. Wounds and Injuries–
nursing.   3. Wounds and Injuries–therapy.   4. Emergency Nursing–
methods.   5. Nursing Assessment–methods. WY 154 T7765 2009]
    RD93.95.T68 2009
    617.1–dc22
                                 2008013073

A catalogue record for this book is available from the British Library.

Set in 9.5 on 11.5 pt Palatino by
SNP Best-set Typesetter Ltd., Hong Kong
Printed and bound in Malaysia by KHL Printing Co Sdn Bhd
1   2009

Contents

Contributors

Elaine Cole, Senior Lecturer ED/Trauma Care, City University/Barts and the London NHS Trust

Joanna Hall, Lecturer Practitioner Paediatric ED, Barts and the London NHS Trust/City University

Antonia Lynch, Consultant Nurse ED, Barts and the London NHS Trust/City University

Sandi Meisner, Senior Coroners Officer, Westminster

Tanya Middlehurst, Senior Nurse, Homerton University Hospital NHS Trust

Foreword

Working at the UK's busiest trauma centre has given Elaine Cole a unique exposure and perspective on the disease of trauma. Her passion for, and commitment to, this complex group of patients is obvious to those who have worked with her and is distilled in this text for those who haven't.

Much is written about the trauma patient and often in reference format, however little is honed from and focused on UK practice. Elaine has successfully bridged this gap with a book that will prove invaluable for all healthcare professionals and students charged with caring for the multiply injured patient.

The style of the text reflects Elaine's and her co-contributors' training in healthcare education. Drawing the content from well referenced material the reader is provided with absolute clarity on the important issues, with learning objectives clearly defined and key information summarised at the end of chapters. The text is peppered with working clinical case studies reminding the reader of the every day practical application of the content.

The best performing centres in the world deliver clinical excellence in trauma not because they have unique treatment modalities or equipment but because they deliver the most basic of care in a quality assured manner with exquisite attention to detail, exactly what this book expounds.

It is with great pleasure that I commend this book to the trauma enthusiast from any background.

Dr Gareth Davies
Clinical Director of HEMS
Consultant in Pre Hospital Care and Emergency Medicine
Barts and the London NHS Trust, UK

Preface

Welcome to the first edition of *Trauma Care: initial assessment and management in the emergency department.* Trauma continues to be a leading cause of death and disability in all age groups, especially the young. In November 2007 the National Confidential Enquiry into Patient Outcome and Death (NCEPOD) launched *Trauma: who cares?* This study has reported that nearly 50% of severely injured patients in the UK did not receive good quality care. Deficiencies in organisational and clinical aspects of trauma care were identified and NCEPOD have called for significant improvements in pre-hospital and in-hospital trauma care.

Practitioners working in these fields must have the knowledge and skills necessary to perform timely assessment and resuscitation for the trauma patient. Early recognition of problems and prompt access to expert help are essential to ensure the best outcomes for the trauma patient.

This book provides the practitioner with a systematic and comprehensive approach to the initial assessment and management of the trauma patient. I hope that pre-hospital and emergency trauma practitioners will find it an invaluable clinical resource.

Elaine Cole
January 2008

Acknowledgements

The editor would like to acknowledge the following people for their help in producing this book: Jo Hall, Toni Lynch, Sandi Meisner and Tanya Middlehurst for sharing their expertise in writing their individual chapters; Dr Helen Cugnoni consultant in emergency medicine for being a critical reader; Tom Cole and Laurence Matthews for their help with the illustrations; Jeff Cole and Mel Armstrong for their help with the photography; Mr Karim Brohi, *Wiley-Blackwell* and the *Spinal Injuries Association* for granting permission to reproduce material in this book; Magenta Lampson at Wiley-Blackwell for her support and advice.

Mechanism of Injury

1

Tanya Middlehurst

INTRODUCTION

Information about the Mechanism of Injury (MOI) can help identify up to 90% of a patient's injuries[1] and give the trauma team an accurate picture of what injuries the patient may have sustained. For the traumatised patient, the importance of such knowledge cannot be underestimated, as an accurate MOI can reduce morbidity and mortality.

Information about the MOI can be gained from the patient where appropriate, from witnesses or from the Emergency Services. However although determining the MOI is an integral part of the initial patient assessment, if the information is not available this should never delay the primary survey and the detection of life-threatening injuries.

The aim of this chapter is to identify the common MOIs that cause traumatic injury and how knowledge of this can assist in the assessment and resuscitation of the trauma patient.

LEARNING OBJECTIVES

At the end of this chapter the reader will be able to:

❏ Understand the principles of energy transmission
❏ Understand the difference between blunt, penetrating and blast trauma
❏ Demonstrate how to relate specific MOIs to certain injury patterns
❏ Understand the importance of MOI in the assessment, management and ongoing evaluation of the trauma patient
❏ Identify trauma scoring systems.

MECHANISM OF INJURY – AN OVERVIEW

Trauma is the leading cause of death in this country under the age of 40 and its effects on society are huge.[2] Disabilities caused by traumatic injuries lead to huge costs for the NHS, through the need to treat and rehabilitate patients, and to employers, who lose working hours and may then need to support an individual's return to work.

In addition there is usually a huge emotional and physical burden placed on the patients themselves, their families and friends, which can be devastating and far-reaching.

Mechanism of injury can be divided into four kinds:[2]

- Blunt
- Penetrating
- Blast
- Thermal.

98% of the trauma in the UK is blunt injury, and other mechanisms make up the rest. Thermal trauma is covered in chapter on burns (see Chapter 9).

The injury that a patient sustains is dependent on several factors: most importantly, it depends on the amount of *energy transmission* that has taken place. Surface area and tissue elasticity are also factors to take into consideration and these will be discussed later in this chapter.

The transmission of energy is sometimes known as velocity or impact energy.

Energy transmission can be considered as a shock wave that moves at various speeds. Energy is carried at the front of the wave and is concentrated in a small space.[1] Energy cannot suddenly disappear, it has to decrease, usually by being absorbed by something else.

Consider a car accident: a car travelling at 40 mph contains a considerable amount of energy. If the car stops suddenly, during a collision with another vehicle for example, the energy will dissipate through the car, and some of this may be transferred to the occupants, potentially causing injury to tissues, organs and bones.

Alternatively think of a bullet: when it is fired from a gun it leaves the barrel at a very high speed. As it travels through the air it will lose energy but if it enters a body there may still be sufficient energy to cause damage, as the body absorbs the rest of the energy.

Injuries caused as a result of energy exchange do not always manifest themselves immediately, so it is important that evaluation is ongoing, so injuries which may appear more slowly can be anticipated and dealt with.

PRE-HOSPITAL INFORMATION

The Emergency Services can be invaluable in providing information about the MOI and about any physical evidence at the scene. A summary of information which may be helpful for the assessment of the patient can be found in Table 1.1.

Occasionally there may be no obvious injury to the patient which can make assessment difficult. However, if the Emergency Services have said there is strong evidence of significant transfer of energy, the patient should always undergo a detailed assessment.

As this chapter will illustrate, certain MOIs can be predictive of serious injury and for pre-hospital personnel there are criteria for alerting the receiving hospital.[2] These criteria can also be used by the emergency department (ED) if a patient arrives via means other then the Emergency Services and a typical list of this type of criteria can be seen in Box 1.1.

BLUNT TRAUMA

Blunt trauma is the most common MOI in most parts of the UK[2] and is the result of energy transfer leading to tissue compression.[3] Blunt trauma is sustained through the following types of incidents:

1. Road Traffic Accidents (RTAs) with the patient in the vehicle
2. Pedestrian impact
3. Cycle and motorcycle accidents

Table 1.1 Pre-hospital information required

Type of event, e.g. RTA with frontal impact, fall, penetrating injury	To understand the basic mechanism
Estimation of energy exchange, e.g. speed of vehicle, distance of fall	To consider the potential for significant injury
What was involved in the impact, e.g. car, tree, concrete, knife	To understand the type of injuries present, e.g. a knife will produce low impact injuries but a gun will produce medium–high impact injuries. A fall onto concrete can produce significant high impact musculoskeletal and organ injury
Were there any clues at the scene?	Some information can be very helpful, e.g. a deformed steering wheel can indicate chest impact, and a bulls-eye break in the windscreen can suggest a head or cervical spine injury. Both suggest significant energy transfer
If drugs or alcohol were known to be involved	To be aware that the patient may still be under the influence of these, which can make assessment more difficult
Past medical history (PMH) and events immediately before the accident	To determine if there was a medical event prior to the incident
Treatment at scene	To help inform ongoing management in the ED
Patient status since incident	To understand how the patient responded to any treatment given and if there is any improvement or deterioration in their condition

4. Assaults
5. Falls.

1. Road Traffic Accidents (RTAs)

When a car comes to a stop, the energy from the moving vehicle will be transferred to the vehicle itself, and then in turn to the occupants. If deceleration (slowing down) takes place slowly, such as over a longer distance, injuries can be less severe. However, deceleration forces, and therefore significant injury, can be much greater if the vehicle comes to a sudden

> **Box 1.1 Mechanisms of injury which suggest the potential for serious injury**
> - Fall of >6 m
> - Pedestrian or cyclist hit by a car
> - Death of other occupant in the same vehicle
> - Ejection from the vehicle/bike
> - Major vehicle deformity or significant intrusion into the passenger space
> - Extrication time >20 min
> - Vehicle rollover
> - Penetrating injury to head or torso
> - All shotgun wounds

stop.[3] This is because the energy level, or velocity, exceeds the tolerance level of the tissue. This leads to tissue disruption and injury.[1]

The nature of the materials involved in the collision and the way in which the energy is dispersed is significant.[3] Modern vehicles are fitted with impact or 'crumple' zones at the front and back which collapse progressively, to absorb as much impact as possible and keep the energy away from the occupants.[3] Larger vehicles tend to be safer than smaller ones. However, regardless of safety features, any significant transfer of energy puts the occupant at risk of serious injury.

RTAs can be categorised according to the type of impact (Box 1.2). The sub-category refers to the nature of the injury that the patient sustains, i.e. *occupant collision* indicates a collision between the occupant and the inside of the vehicle, or outside if they are ejected; and *organ collision* indicates the impact between the patient's organs and the internal framework of the body. Some patients can suffer both.

Occupant collision: frontal impact

A frontal impact is a collision with an object in front of the vehicle, which suddenly reduces its speed.[1] It accounts for the majority of injuries and deaths sustained in RTAs. As the

---

Box 1.2 Categories of road traffic accident

Occupant collision

Frontal
Lateral
Rear
Rollover
Ejection

Organ collision

Compression injury
Declaration injury
Restraint injury

---

vehicle comes to a stop the occupant(s) continue to move forward with the same speed as the vehicle, until something stops them.[1] This could be the steering wheel, dashboard, windscreen, or ground if the occupant is ejected. Frontal impacts cause shortening of the car as the bonnet caves in and the engine and dashboard are forced backwards into the passenger compartment.[2] Any such deformity of the passenger compartment indicates a significant impact.[3]

In this type of impact, lower limb injuries are common as they get trapped by the engine and dashboard, or impact against pedals.[2] The occupant hitting the steering wheel can result in blunt torso injuries to structures such as the liver, spleen and stomach, as well as fractured ribs, sternum and flail chest. Finally head, face and cervical spine injuries can result from impact against the steering wheel or windscreen.

The occupant can also follow a *down and under* pathway, whereby they slide under the dashboard.[1] This can lead to fractures and dislocations of the ankle, knee, femur and femoral head.[1,3]

Rear passengers can sustain injuries as well, especially if unrestrained. Any unrestrained passenger can sustain severe facial injuries from being thrown forward. In addition front seat passengers are at risk of being injured by unrestrained rear passengers who are thrust forward.

Occupant collision: lateral impact

A lateral impact occurs when a vehicle is hit from the side and the occupant is accelerated away from the point of impact. Lateral impact RTAs are second only to frontal impacts in terms of injury and death,[1] and 75% of victims of lateral impacts are over the age of 50.

Case study 1.1 Lateral impact injuries

A 75-year-old man is pulling out of a side street in his car and is hit on the driver's side by a car estimated to be travelling at 35 mph. According to witnesses he was unconscious for a period of 2–3 minutes. At the scene it is noted that there is a crack through the window on the driver's door.

On arrival to the ED the Emergency Services report that he was conscious on their arrival but complaining of right-sided abdominal and chest pain, as well as neck pain and right upper arm pain. He has a large boggy wound on the right side of his head, an increased respiratory rate (RR) and tenderness on the right side of his chest. His right upper arm is bruised and swollen.

Injuries will relate to which side the force was applied, so a lateral impact to the driver's side could potentially result in injuries to the right side of the body, such as a liver laceration, whereas a left-sided impact may result in a passenger sustaining a ruptured spleen.

Victims can also sustain lateral flail chest injuries, pulmonary contusion and kidney injury. If the force is significant enough the occupant may be pushed from one side of the car to another, leading to injuries on both sides. The head can also be injured if the victim strikes another occupant of the vehicle or hits their head on the window the same side as the collision.[3]

A lateral impact may also cause upper and lower musculoskeletal injuries, typically fractures to the pelvis, ribs and upper arm, with associated internal injuries.[2] Neck injuries can occur in addition, as a result of a lateral impact.

Occupant collision: rear impact

These impacts differ from frontal and lateral impacts, as they often occur when the vehicle involved is already stationary, and is struck from behind. However, like a lateral impact, the occupant is accelerated forward due to the energy transfer from behind.[1] This may subsequently lead to the vehicle being propelled forward leading to an additional frontal impact.

Injuries that occur in this type of impact are predominantly whiplash injuries, caused by hyperextension of the neck and often exacerbated by a poorly functioning head-rest.[1,4] Fractures of the cervical spine can also occur.

Occupant collision: rollover

When a car rolls over the energy can be dissipated over a long distance, which can sometimes minimise injury to the occupants, particularly if they are restrained.[3,4] However, the chaotic and multiple movements sustained in a rollover can and do cause significant injury and these should always be excluded.

During a rollover, injury severity can depend on whether the occupant was restrained or unrestrained. An unrestrained occupant can impact on any part of the vehicle interior[1] or could be ejected.[4] Musculoskeletal injuries to any part of the body may occur, with associated internal organ damage.

Roof collapse can lead to significant head injury[4] and compression fractures of the spine are common. Figure 1.1 illustrates a rollover with extensive roof damage.

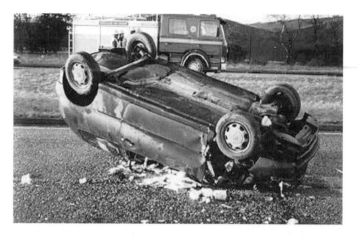

Fig. 1.1 Vehicle rollover RTA. (Permission given by K Brohi. Source www. trauma.org)

Occupant collision: ejection

If the patient is ejected from the vehicle, the likelihood of serious injury increases by 300%[1,4] as there has been sufficient energy transfer to force them from the vehicle and they will have hit the ground at considerable speed.[2] Anyone else in the vehicle that has not been ejected may still have been subjected to severe energy force.

Organ collision: compression injury

Compression injuries occur when the anterior (front) part of the torso stops moving forwards and the posterior (back) portion of the torso and internal organs continue to move forward. This leads to compression of the organs from the posterior part of the internal chest and abdomen,[1] but can also occur inside the skull causing brain injury.[3]

Examples of compression injuries include:

- Blunt myocardial injury
- Lung contusion
- Flail chest

9

- Pneumothorax
- Bowel injury.

Organ collision: deceleration injury

These injuries occur when a vehicle or person comes to a sudden halt, after moving at speed.[3] When the body stops moving forwards the stabilising part of an organ also stops moving, but the organ itself continues to do so. This can lead to a shearing force which can detach the stabilising structure from its organ.

Examples of this type of injury are to the kidney and spleen, which both shear away from their respective pedicles. In the brain, the posterior part of the brain separates from the skull, tearing vessels in the process,[1] leading to cerebral contusion.[3] The aorta can rupture in a high speed RTA, where deceleration leads to the aortic arch shearing off from the descending aorta, an injury which is usually fatal in seconds.[2]

Organ collision: restraint injury

The use of three-point restraint seat belts has been shown to reduce death in RTAs by up to 70%.[1] However, if used incorrectly, and sometimes when used correctly, injuries can occur.

To function correctly the lap portion of the seat belt must be below the anterior/superior iliac spines and above the femur,[1] and must be tight enough to remain in place during any impact.

If it is worn incorrectly, such as too high, then the forward motion of the posterior abdominal wall and spine can trap organs such as liver, pancreas, spleen or kidney against the belt at the front. This can result in burst injuries and lacerations to these organs[1] such as duodenal rupture.[2] The shoulder portion of a seat belt can cause neck injury if worn too high.[3]

Even when a belt is applied correctly the energy exchange can be sufficient to lead to injuries such as:

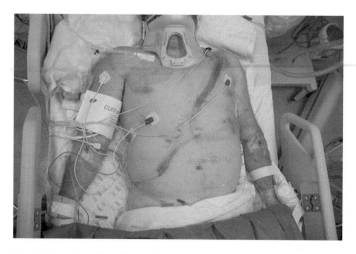

Fig. 1.2 Restraint injury. (Permission given by K Brohi. Source www.trauma. org)

- Fractures of the clavicle
- Cardiac contusions
- Pneumothorax
- Rib and sternal fractures.

Pattern bruising over the abdomen or chest from a seat belt suggests significant energy exchange and the trauma team should be suspicious of associated internal injury[2] (Figure 1.2).

Availability of airbags in vehicles may reduce injuries in frontal impacts, and side impacts.[1,4] They work by spreading the deceleration forces over a large area and so reduce forward movement and impact.[3] However, they provide no protection in rollovers or rear impact and can actually cause injury to patients who are not in the usual position, such as facing backwards when the airbag is set off.[4] Once activated airbags can cause friction and heat burns.[3]

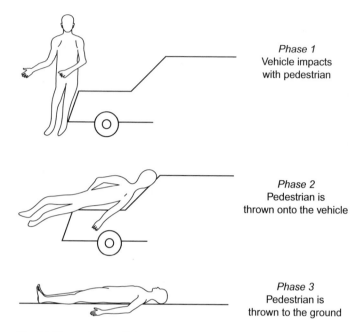

Phase 1
Vehicle impacts
with pedestrian

Phase 2
Pedestrian is
thrown onto the vehicle

Phase 3
Pedestrian is
thrown to the ground

Fig. 1.3 Three phases of injury

2. Pedestrian impact

Pedestrian injuries are primarily urban in nature and children make up a large proportion of those killed or injured every year.[1] The type of injuries seen in pedestrian impact are predominantly thoracic, head and lower extremity, due to the three-phase nature of the impact involved in a pedestrian incident (Figure 1.3).

These three phases consist of:

1. The *vehicle-bumper* impact
2. The *vehicle bonnet and/or windscreen* impact
3. The *ground* impact.

Injuries sustained during the vehicle-bumper impact will vary with the height of the victim; in an adult the impact would normally be against the legs and pelvis[1] whereas a child may sustain blunt chest and abdominal injuries. Different types of vehicles, such as lower riding sports cars, or higher four wheel drive vehicles, will also alter the impact point. Information about the type of vehicle is helpful in determining probable injury patterns. If a patient is hit by a bus or lorry, they may either be thrown to the side of the vehicle or dragged under.[2] This can result in any part of the body being run over or dragged along beneath a vehicle.

After the victim has hit the bumper, they may then be thrown onto the bonnet and can impact with the windscreen as well.[1,4] Occasionally patients may be thrown over the roof of the car, if the impact is great enough.[2] Types of injures sustained during this phase will be dependent on which part of the body impacts with the car, and at what speed the incident occurred at.

Finally the victim will fall from the bonnet (or roof if the speed was great enough), and impact with the ground. This will typically cause head and neck injuries as the victim falls to the ground. Organ compression can also occur as the patient comes to a stop.[1] At this point the patient may also be at risk from being run over by other vehicles in the road.

Running-over injuries occur when the vehicle, or part of the vehicle, goes over the victim or may even drag them along the road. Severe injuries can occur to any part of the body[3] and these are often immediately life threatening.

Due to the lower point of impact, children may be prone to being thrown to the side or under the vehicle,[2] although they too can be forced onto the bonnet if conditions are right. Children will often turn to face the car before impact, thereby turning the impact into a frontal one,[2] whereas adults tend to turn away.[3]

3. Cycle and motorcycle accidents

Cyclists and motorcyclists (and their passengers) may sustain compression, acceleration and deceleration, and shearing injuries.[1] Motorcyclists are afforded some protection if they are wearing appropriate clothing, such as leathers, boots and gloves, and there is a legal requirement for motorcyclists to wear a helmet. Despite this most motorcycle deaths are as a result of head injuries.[3] Tight leather trousers, such as those worn by motorcyclists, can help to reduce blood loss in lower limb fractures.[3]

Cyclists however may have a lot less protection and despite the evidence showing that helmets reduce the incidence of head injury by 85%,[1] there is no legal requirement to wear one.

For cyclists and motorcyclists, there are common MOIs which can predict injury patterns, although injuries can be more severe for motorcyclists due to the speeds involved.[2]

In a frontal impact the front wheel of the cycle/motorcycle collides with an object and stops. The rider, however, will continue to move forward until something stops this momentum, such as the ground or another stationary object.[1] During this event, the head, chest or abdomen can impact with the handlebars leading to blunt trauma to these areas, such as pelvic fractures and injuries to the organs contained within.

If the cyclist is ejected from the bike, femoral injuries may occur as a result of impact with the handlebars.[1] The final impact, with the ground, can result in other injuries such as spinal fractures.

If the cyclist is hit from the side, they may sustain open or closed fractures, or crush injuries, to the lower limbs[1] as well as ejection and ground-impact injuries as described above. Ejection from the bike may also lead to the patient being involved in a further incident with another vehicle. Friction burns may occur as the victim slides along the ground.[3]

Another common MOI with cyclists is known as 'laying the bike down': to avoid being trapped between their cycle/motorcycle and another object, the cyclist may turn the bike sideways and drop the bike and inside leg onto the ground,[1] in order to slow themselves down. This can lead to significant fractures and/or soft tissue injury to the lower limbs.

4. Assaults

Victims of assaults are most commonly young males[4] and alcohol is often involved. Injuries sustained during an assault will vary according to the force and instruments used. A minor blow to the head can produce a scalp haematoma or wound, whereas a harder blow can lead to a skull fracture, cerebral contusions and extra- or subdural haematomas.[2]

Commonly defensive injuries may be present, such as trauma to the limbs, hands and back,[2] where the person has tried to protect themselves. Head and facial injuries are also common and a victim that has been kicked or stamped on whilst on the ground may also sustain significant injuries to their torso.[4]

5. Falls

Falls predominantly affect the under-5 and over-60 age groups. They produce injury through deceleration and the severity of injuries depends on several factors:

- The *height* of the fall and therefore the speed of impact
- The contact *surface* that the victim lands on
- The *position* on impact.

The greater the height, the greater the velocity and so the greater the deceleration when the victim comes to a stop.[3] As a general guide, falls from three times the height of the victim result in serious injury such as those described in the deceleration section above.

If the surface that stops the fall is hard, such as concrete, the injuries can be more severe as the rate of deceleration is increased[1] and all the energy is transferred to the body.[4] This can result in compression injuries as described earlier.

Although the information is not always available, the position of the body on impact can also help to determine the nature of injuries that the patient may sustain. In a fall if someone lands on their feet, energy will be transferred via the bones of the lower limbs to the pelvis and then the spine, resulting in calcaneal and femoral neck fractures and injuries to the vertebra.[1] If the person lands on their back, energy transfer takes place over a wider area and so tissue damage may be less severe.

In the older person co-morbid conditions should be considered, such as heart disease or chronic respiratory problems, which may have contributed to the fall.[4]

PENETRATING INJURIES

Penetrating injuries constitute gunshot wounds, stab wounds and impalements.

The severity of injury will depend on the velocity of the penetrating force:

- Stab wounds are low velocity
- Handguns are medium velocity
- Military rifles and shotguns are high velocity.

The velocity of an impalement injury will depend on how it was caused, but are usually low to medium energy.

The same principles of energy transmission occur with penetrating wounds, as with all other types of trauma. However, in penetrating wounds it is discussed in terms of cavitation.

Cavitation

Cavitation occurs when an object, such as a bullet or knife, collides with tissues. At the point of collision the tissues move away from the object causing a cavity. The amount of cavitation produced is directly proportional to the amount of energy transferred and will also depend on the density of the tissues, the size of the front aspect of the penetrating object and the elasticity of the tissues.[3] In penetrating trauma there is both temporary and permanent cavitation.

Gunshot wounds

Gunshot wounds are medium or high velocity and the severity of the injury largely depends on what the velocity is, as this dictates how much energy is transferred to the tissues.[2] In a penetrating injury, this energy will form a cavity, as described above, and the characteristics of this cavity will influence any subsequent injury.[5]

High energy weapons such as hunting rifles and assault weapons generally cause much greater damage because they create much larger cavities,[3] extending far beyond the track of the bullet. These blasts can carry clothing and debris into the wound, by creating a temporary vacuum which sucks detritus into the wound.[2] This can result in infection if the debris is not removed.[1]

High velocity wounds can be lethal at close range although injury becomes less severe as the distance between the gun and victim increases.[1] Information about how close the firearm was when it was discharged can therefore be helpful. However, the majority of shootings take place at close range with handguns, and so the potential for severe injury is significant.[3]

Medium velocity wounds such as those from handguns do not usually produce extensive cavitation.[2]

The amount of tissue damage will also be influenced by the density and elasticity of the tissues involved. A bullet from a firearm will dissipate a huge amount of energy to the tissues and in general the denser the tissue the greater amount of energy transferred, and the greater degree of damage.[5]

Solid organs such as the brain and liver are surrounded by a rigid or semi-rigid casing and have very little elasticity and so absorb a lot of energy[2] leading to devastating injuries. Bones, which also have no elastic recoil may shatter on impact whereas the lungs, which are less dense and more elastic, are less likely to be affected by cavitation as they absorb less energy.[2]

Some bullets are designed to increase the amount of damage they cause[1] by flattening, fragmenting or exploding on impact, to increase the amount of cavitation and tissue damage.[2] If the velocity is high enough, the resulting cavity can be up to 30 times the diameter of the bullet.[1]

As well as an entrance wound, there may also be an exit wound. Depending on the velocity and site of entry, the missile will follow the path of least resistance and may exit the body.[1] Entrance wounds may have powder burns or tattooing around the edges and exit wounds tend to be ragged.[1] There can be multiple exit wounds.[3]

The presence of two wounds however does not always indicate an entrance and exit, but may in fact be two entrance wounds, with bullets still in situ.[1] Estimating the path of the bullet should not take precedence over assessing and stabilising the patient.

Stab wounds

These low energy wounds cause direct tissue damage along a straight track[2] and knives are the commonest instrument used. If a weapon remains in the body it should be left until it can be safely removed by a senior surgeon. This should be carried out in a resuscitation setting or theatres as removal may cause haemorrhage to occur.[2]

Case study 1.2 Penetrating injury

A man is his early twenties is brought to the ED by a group of friends. He has been involved in a fight and has blood on his face and shirt. He is taken to the resuscitation room for assessment. The nurse notes that he has a number of slash wounds to his face, hands and wrists, although these are not actively bleeding. After getting the patient undressed a small stab wound is located beneath his right armpit measuring 1 cm in length. Despite this seemingly small injury the nurse notes that the patient looks pale, has difficulty in taking deep breaths and is tachycardic with a pulse of 118. The trauma team is immediately summoned.

A patient who has been stabbed may only appear to have a small wound but this will initially be of unknown length and so should be subject to careful assessment.[5] 25% of penetrating abdominal injuries also involve the thorax as well and should be assessed to exclude such injuries.[3] Wounds to the chest below the nipple line may also involve the abdomen.

If the information is available, it can be useful to know if the assailant was male or female, as men tend to stab upwards and women tend to stab downwards. This can be useful in trying to determine the path of the knife and the possible injuries.

Impalements

These are predominantly accidental and often involve a larger object than a knife,[5] such as machinery, a fence post or railings. Victims of impalements may need to be assessed with the object still in situ. Like stab wounds, if the impaling object is still in situ it should only be removed after careful assessment: more often than not this is in an operating theatre.

BLAST INJURIES

Explosions have the potential to cause multi-system, life-threatening injuries in one or more victims and need careful assessment and management.[6] More recently the need to also screen for signs of radiation and/or chemical contamination of the patient has been highlighted. Such patients may require specialist decontamination at the scene of the blast or on arrival at the ED.

In a blast there is a huge release of energy, known as a shock front or blast front, which spreads out rapidly and will cause damage to whatever is in its path, whether this is people or buildings. The further away from the centre of the explosion the shock front travels, the less energy it carries with it.[2]

Blast injuries are classified as:

- Primary
- Secondary
- Tertiary.

Primary blast injuries

These injuries result from the direct effects of the pressure wave and are most damaging to air-containing organs such as the eardrum (tympanum), lungs and gut.[1] Bruising, oedema and rupture of lung tissue, sometimes leading to pneumothorax, can occur[1,2] and the alveoli and pulmonary veins may also be ruptured, leading to potential air embolism. Intraocular haemorrhage, as well as retinal disruption, may be present and intestinal rupture can also occur.[1]

The tympanic membranes may rupture and presence of this injury suggests that significant exposure has occurred,[2] and although serious injury may not be present, it should nevertheless be excluded. Evidence of tympanic membrane rupture should lead to the patient having a chest x-ray to exclude chest injury such as pulmonary contusion.

It should also be remembered that absence of this injury does not preclude the presence of other serious injuries. Patients with these injuries are usually suffering from temporary hearing loss and so communication can be difficult.

Secondary blast injuries

These result from flying objects, disturbed as a result of the blast, hitting the patient. Depending on the nature, location and force of the blast, these may be a combination of blunt and penetrating injuries to any part of the body.

Tertiary blast injuries

These occur when the patient is lifted and thrown by the force of the blast, and are sustained when they impact against something, such as a wall or the ground. Again this may cause both blunt and penetrating injuries depending on the nature of the blast. They are characteristic of high energy explosions[6] and traumatic amputations are common.

INJURY SCORING SYSTEMS

Injury scoring systems are used to determine the potential for someone having sustained a serious injury.[7,8] They are useful in situations where there is more than one casualty, as they allow Emergency Services and ED personnel to prioritise the

---

Box 1.3 Injury scoring systems

The Injury Severity Score (ISS) is one of the most widely used and is an anatomical system which provides an overall score for each patient. Patients are given a score for each injury related to one of six body regions:

- Head
- Face
- Chest
- Abdomen
- Extremities
- External

The highest score for each region is squared and added together to produce the ISS score

The Revised Trauma Score (RTS) is a scoring system based on the physiological signs of the patient. Scores are given for the first set of readings of:

- Glasgow Coma Scale (GCS)
- Systolic BP
- Respiratory rate

The totals are added together and the lower the score, the more seriously injured the patient is

The Abbreviated Injury Score (AIS) scores injuries from 1 (minor) to 6 (fatal)

---

more severely injured patients.[7-9] Commonly used scoring systems include (Box 1.3):

- The Injury Severity Score (ISS)
- The Abbreviated Injury Score (AIS)
- The Revised Trauma Score (RTS).

To assist in calculations of the scores, the Trauma Injury Severity Score (TRISS) calculator determines the probability of survival from the ISS, RTS and the patient's age.[10]

CONCLUSION

Mechanism of traumatic injury can be categorised as blunt, penetrating and blast and each will produce distinct injury patterns. An awareness of the mechanism of injury a patient may have sustained, as well as detailed assessment in the ED, can be invaluable in helping to predict the nature and severity of their injuries. This in turn can reduce morbidity and mortality.

KEY INFORMATION BOX

- Pre-hospital information about the scene of the incident can indicate potential injuries
- A significant mechanism of injury should cause a high index of suspicion
- Injury can be caused by force from outside of and within the body
- A fatality at the scene is predictive of severe force
- Penetrating injuries may seem innocuous but there may be significant damage beneath the wound
- Primary blast injuries may cause deafness due to ruptured tympanic membranes – this can be indicative of lung and gut injuries
- Injury scoring systems can help predict injury severity, morbidity and mortality in a single or group of patients.

REFERENCES

1. American College of Surgeons (2004) Biomechanics of injury. In: Advanced trauma life support for doctors. Student course manual (7th edn), 315–335. American College of Surgeons, Chicago
2. Greaves I, Porter KM, Ryan JM (Eds) (2001) Mechanism of injury. In: Trauma care manual, 99–114. Arnold, London
3. Eaton J (2005) Kinetics and mechanics of injury. In: Principles and practice of trauma nursing (Ed O'Shea R), 15–35. Elsevier, Edinburgh

4. Grossman MD (2002) Patterns of blunt injury. In: The trauma manual (2nd edn) (Eds Peitzman AB, Rhodes M, Schwab CW, Yealy DM, Fabian TC), 4–9. Lippincott, Williams & Wilkins, Philadelphia

5. DiGiacomo JC, Reilly JF (2002) Mechanisms of injury/penetrating trauma. In: The trauma manual (2nd edn) (Eds Peitzman AB, Rhodes M, Schwab CW, Yealy DM, Fabian TC), 10–16. Lippincott, Williams & Wilkins, Philadelphia

6. Lavonas E, Pennardt A (2006) Blast injuries. http://www.emedicine.com/emerg/topic63.htm

7. Dillon B, Wang W, Bouarma O (2006) A comparison study of the injury score models. European Journal of Trauma and Emergency Surgery 32:538–547

8. Brohi K (2007) Injury severity score. http://www.trauma.org/index.php/main/article/383

9. Brohi K (2007) Revised trauma score. http://www.trauma.org/index.php/main/article/386

10. Brohi K (2007) TRISS: Trauma – Injury Severity Score http://www.trauma.org/index.php/main/article/387/

2 | Initial Assessment and Resuscitation of the Trauma Patient

Elaine Cole

INTRODUCTION

Traumatic injury is the leading cause of death and disability in people aged between 1 and 40 years in the developed world[1,2] and after heart disease and cancer, a common cause of death in the older population.[3] A percentage of trauma deaths have been shown to be preventable,[2] with new vehicles manufactured to increase safety, the existence of injury prevention campaigns and injury minimisation programmes. However, in the UK 240 people are severely injured each week,[4] resulting in 3400 deaths per year.[1] Therefore, it is essential that frontline staff who work with trauma patients are educated and updated in the care and management of injuries, to ensure the best outcome for the patient.[4]

The initial assessment and resuscitation of a trauma patient may happen in the pre-hospital field by one or two people, or in the emergency department (ED) by a small or large team, dependent on available resources. Regardless of where it happens or by whom, the goal of early trauma care is to *assess, diagnose and simultaneously address life-threatening problems which can cause death or serious morbidity.*[5]

The aim of this chapter is to understand the principles of systematic assessment, resuscitation and stabilisation of the trauma patient in the early stages of care.

LEARNING OBJECTIVES

By the end of this chapter the reader will be able to:

❏ Define a trauma team and trauma team roles
❏ Describe initial assessment priorities in relation to ABCDE
❏ Understand each stage of the primary survey
❏ Identify the components of the secondary survey.

TRAUMA CARE IN THE ED

The guidelines for the initial assessment and resuscitation of traumatically injured patients devised by the American College of Surgeons[3] are followed internationally. The 'Advanced Trauma Life Support' course (ATLS) teaches doctors how to assess and treat patients in the early stages of trauma care and courses using similar guidelines have been adapted for nurses and paramedics.[2]

The American College of Surgeons describe a trimodal death distribution, where death from trauma occurs in 1 of 3 time periods:[5]

• First – within seconds or minutes of the injury
• Second – within minutes to hours following the injury
• Third – several days or weeks following the injury.

Principles from ATLS focus on the assessment and resuscitation during the second time period. In this phase, injuries that cause hypoxia, hypovolaemia or a rapidly accumulating brain haemorrhage need prompt recognition and treatment.[6] This is important not only in relation to patient survival in the ED but also survival in the third phase of care. Delayed treatment of hypoxia or haemorrhage will result in complex problems such as acidosis and coagulopathy (clotting derangement)[7] when the patient is in intensive care (ICU) or the trauma ward.

In order to recognise life-threatening problems and initiate prompt treatment, a systematic approach to assessment is necessary. ED staff need to identify signs and symptoms that are suggestive of a serious injury and access expert help and intervention quickly. In many EDs this means activation of a consultant-led multidisciplinary trauma team with skilled personnel who have the pre-requisite knowledge and skills.[2,4]

The trauma team

The trauma team should be made up of clinicians who carry out pre-assigned roles so that several interventions can occur simultaneously.[3] Membership of the trauma team is dependent on the institution and the resources available, as are the team roles and responsibilities. Box 2.1 shows an example of trauma team roles. Most trauma teams in the UK consist of doctors, nurses, radiographers and other practitioners, who should have received training in trauma management

---

Box 2.1 Trauma team roles

Team leader – Consultant (ED or trauma surgeon)
Anaesthetist – Specialist registrar grade or above, to manage the airway with cervical spine control
Trauma surgeon – Specialist registrar or above, to perform the primary assessment, FAST scan and initial surgical consult
Junior ED doctor – to assist with procedures, establish venous access, take blood
Nurse 1 – trauma trained nurse to liaise with team leader, supports nurse 2, provides analgesia, liaises with family
Nurse 2 – to assist trauma surgeon and anaesthetist
Operating department practitioner – to assist anaesthetist
Radiographer – to perform imaging
Radiologist – to interpret imaging
Scribe – to document findings and interventions (this role may be a nurse or a doctor depending on the institution)
Neurosurgeon and orthopaedic surgeon – available for opinion during the trauma call

---

to ensure the appropriate level of clinical knowledge and skills.

Human factors and the trauma team

As well as clinical competence, human factors, i.e. non-technical skills, are an essential component of effective team working.[3] This includes:

- A defined leader trained in team management
- Clear organisation and role definition
- Effective communication strategies
- Situational awareness of 'the bigger picture'
- An opportunity to brief prior to the patient's arrival
- An opportunity to debrief after the trauma call.

Contemporary trauma education programmes should include these aspects of trauma care, and whilst many trauma courses are aimed at nurses or doctors, multi-professional trauma team training would enhance team working.[3]

Trauma team activation

Case study 2.1 Trauma team activation

The ambulance service ring the ED with a priority call. They are at the scene of a road traffic accident where two cars have collided head on. Despite witnesses stating that neither car was going particularly fast, a child has been ejected from one of the vehicles and has been taken to a hospital with a paediatric intensive care unit. The other occupant of the car only appears to have a left knee injury and is cardiovascularly stable. However, the ambulance service have decided this person needs a priority call. The nurse who accepts the call doesn't know whether to activate the trauma team.

Trauma teams are usually alerted following advanced warning information from the pre-hospital care staff. If the mechanism of injury and the status of the patient are suggestive of serious traumatic injury then the trauma team will be alerted (see Table 1.1 and Box 1.1 for more information).

Horizontal vs. vertical assessment of the trauma patient

Assessment of the trauma patient is usually performed in two stages, firstly the primary and later the secondary surveys.[2,5,6] The initial assessment, known as the primary survey, has five components 'A,B,C,D,E':

- Airway with cervical spine control
- Breathing and ventilation
- Circulation and haemorrhage control
- Disability and dysfunction
- Exposure and environmental control.

Horizontal assessment of the patient occurs where there is a trauma team present and each step (A, B, C, D, E) is carried out simultaneously with pre-assigned roles. This is a timely and effective method of rapid assessment and treatment and should be used for all seriously injured patients brought in by pre-hospital personnel.[2,8]

Vertical assessment of the patient occurs where there are one or two people (such as paramedics) assessing A, then B then C and so on in a sequential order.[2] This organisation is not as time efficient and usually takes place in situations where there are fewer people available.

Vertical assessment also occurs in the ED when a patient presents whose injuries are not immediately apparent or the mechanism of injury is not suggestive of anything serious. When conducting a vertical assessment, it is essential that the individual nurse or clinician has the pre-requisite knowledge and skills to do this. It is vital that this individual knows when to ask for expert help or when to activate the trauma team to ensure optimal patient outcome. Box 2.2 suggests criteria for activating the trauma team either before the patient arrives, or following the initial patient assessment.

Box 2.2 Activation of a trauma team

Trauma victims with any of the following:

- Actual or potential airway compromise
- Signs of a pneumothorax (respiratory distress)
- SpO_2 <90%
- Heart rate >100/minutes (adults)
- GCS <14 associated with a head injury
- Penetrating wound anywhere from the neck to the thighs
- Any gunshot wound
- Fall from >25 feet/8 metres
- Ejection from a vehicle

Children involved in a traumatic incident with:

- An altered level of consciousness
- Capillary refill time of >3 seconds
- Tachycardia
- A child who was a pedestrian or cyclist hit by a vehicle

PRIMARY SURVEY: INITIAL ASSESSMENT AND RESUSCITATION

If advanced warning is given and the team are notified before the patient arrives, equipment, resources and staff can be prepared. This includes:

- Hand washing
- Assembly of the trauma team with a briefing by the team leader
- Each team member should wear gloves, protective eye wear and gowns or aprons (plus x-ray lead aprons if available)
- Pre-registration of the patient to allow for ordering of blood tests and blood products and diagnostic imaging
- Reassuring other patients and relatives in the vicinity of where the trauma call will take place.

Airway with cervical spine control

The first step of assessment is to ascertain airway patency.[5] The airway can become obstructed due to structural damage, e.g.

Table 2.1 Systematic airway assessment

1. Talk	If the patient can talk freely the airway is patent
2. Look and listen	For signs of airway obstruction: blood, vomit
3. Open	Chin lift and jaw thrust, NOT HEAD TILT
4. Suction	Use a rigid suction catheter under direct vision
5. Adjuncts	Oropharyngeal or nasopharyngeal airways
6. Definitive airway	Endotracheal intubation or surgical airway

bleeding or swelling of the face, mouth or oropharynx, a reduced level of consciousness or vomiting and aspiration. Expert help should be sought immediately if there is any doubt about the patient's ability to maintain their own airway.

A systematic approach to airway management is essential, as simple manoeuvres may be all that the patient requires to keep the airway patent. Furthermore, ED staff must be able to maintain a patent airway until expert help arrives. Table 2.1 shows the sequential approach to airway assessment.

1. Talk to the patient
Talking to the patient not only establishes psychological support but also assesses the airway.[8] If the patient is talking freely in a normal voice (i.e. no grunting or hoarseness) then it can be assumed that the airway is patent. Talking to the patient throughout the primary survey assessment is recommended to provide support, explain procedures and continually assess the airway.

2. Look and listen for signs of obstruction
If the patient is not able to talk freely, the airway patency is at risk. The practitioner should look and listen for signs of obstruction.

Look in the mouth for:

- Any obstruction/foreign body
- Bleeding
- Swelling
- Burns
- Soft tissue injury.

Listen for:

- Breath sounds from the mouth
- Snoring
- Grunting
- Gurgling
- Stridor – a 'crowing' noise on inspiration
- Hoarseness.

3. Open the airway
Once an airway obstruction has been diagnosed, the airway should be opened immediately. A chin lift or jaw thrust manoeuvre (Figure 2.1) should be used, rather than a head tilt which may worsen a cervical spine injury.

4. Suction
If the obstruction is caused by a foreign body, vomit or bleeding, this should be removed with suction. A wide bore rigid

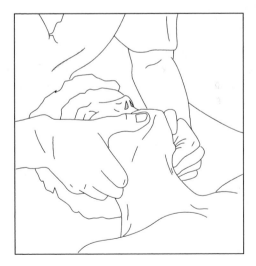

Fig. 2.1 Jaw thrust. (Reproduced with permission from Hodgetts T, Turner L (2006) Trauma rules 2 (2nd edn), figure 16.1. Blackwell Publishing, Oxford)

Yankauer™ suction catheter is recommended. Keep the tip or end of the catheter in direct vision to avoid inserting it too far and causing further damage or stimulating a gag reflex.

5. Insertion of airway adjuncts

If the airway obstruction persists, placement of an artificial airway may help to improve patency. *Airway adjuncts must be used in conjunction with an airway opening manoeuvre as they will not ensure patency on their own in the unconscious patient lying supine.*

The choice of airway is either:

- An oropharyngeal airway (Guedel) in the unconscious patient without a gag reflex[8] OR
- A nasopharyngeal airway if a gag reflex is present.[8]

To ensure the correct size, an oropharyngeal airway is measured from the tragus of the ear to the corner of the mouth (Figure 2.2). It is inserted upside down, rotated 180 degrees and then pushed into position. The flange should sit flush

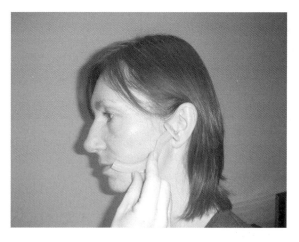

Fig. 2.2 Sizing an oropharyngeal airway

with the lips. *If the patient gags or coughs during insertion the airway should be removed.*

The size of a nasopharyngeal airway is chosen by ensuring that the diameter of the tube is smaller than the diameter of the nostril. The airway should be lubricated prior to introduction and inserted into the nose with a slight twisting motion. Nasopharyngeal airways extend from the nostril to the nasopharynx, with the wider end sitting at the nostril.

Nasopharyngeal airways should not be used for patients with facial injuries or suspected base of skull fractures due to the risk of inserting the airway into the injured area.

6. Definitive airway: intubation

Following steps 1–5 it may be evident that the patient needs a definitive airway secured. This means a tracheal tube securely placed in the trachea, cuffed in an adult, uncuffed in a small child. Intubation should be carried out by a clinician trained in advanced airway management.

Indications for a definitive airway include:[9]

- Apnoea
- Inability to maintain the patient's airway with other means (steps 1–5 described above)
- The need to protect the lungs from aspiration
- Potential airway compromise, e.g. following burns, facial fractures
- GCS < 8
- Inability to maintain adequate oxygenation using a facemask.

Many trauma patient who need to be intubated still have a gag reflex, muscle tone and clenched teeth, hence anaesthesia may be needed.[8] Therefore a rapid sequence induction (RSI) is used, delivering anaesthetic in a safe controlled manner. Three people are needed for an RSI – the clinician to insert the tube, an assistant to perform cricoid pressure (to prevent aspiration of stomach contents into the lungs) and one person to deliver drugs, attach monitoring and observe the patient.

Box 2.3 Equipment for an RSI

- Two laryngoscopes – checked and working
- Suction catheter
- Magill's forceps
- Endotracheal tubes – one a size smaller and one a size larger than the expected size
- Gum elastic bougie or introducer
- 10 ml syringe for cuff inflation
- Catheter mount and filter
- Inflating bag or a bag-valve device
- Oxygen supply
- CO_2 detector or monitoring
- Anaesthetic drugs each drawn up in a syringe clearly labelled
- Intravenous flush

Everyone involved in an RSI should be trained and competent as it is a high risk procedure. The technique is as follows, although local policies may vary slightly:

- Prepare equipment (Box 2.3)
- Attach ECG and oxygen saturation monitoring
- Pre-oxygenate the patient with high flow oxygen
- Assistant stands on the patient's left and applies cricoid pressure as directed by the clinician
- Administer an anaesthetic agent (e.g. etomidate) as per local policy
- Administer a muscle relaxant (e.g. suxamethonium) as per local policy
- A laryngoscope is used to visualise the vocal cords (the trachea is beyond this)
- Insert the endotracheal tube (size appropriate to the patient) – an introducer may be used
- Third person inflates the cuff with air in a 10 ml syringe
- Confirm the procedure by looking at the chest, listening for breath sounds and measuring CO_2

- Release cricoid pressure
- Ventilate the patient.

7. Definitive airway: surgical airway

A surgical airway may be needed if there is severe injury or swelling to the face or oropharynx, and intubation is not possible. There are two types of surgical airway:

- Needle cricothyroidotomy with jet insufflation
- Surgical cricothyroidotomy.

A needle cricothyroidotomy is used in children under the age of 12 (see Chapter 10). A large bore cannula is inserted through the cricothyroid membrane (Figure 2.3), the needle is removed and a Y-connector attached to deliver oxygen at 1 L/min.[9] Intermittent ventilation known as jet insufflation can be achieved by occluding the hole in the Y-connector for 1 second

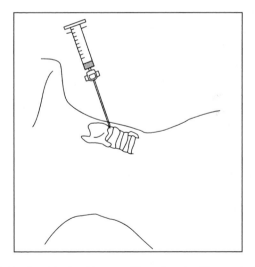

Fig. 2.3 Needle cricothyroidotomy. (Reproduced with permission from Hodgetts T, Turner L (2006) Trauma rules 2 (2nd edn), figure 21.2. Blackwell Publishing, Oxford)

and releasing for 4 seconds.[5] Oxygen can be delivered in this manner for 30–45 minutes, after which time CO_2 levels will have risen and the child urgently requires a definitive airway and ventilation.

A surgical cricothyroidotomy requires a surgical incision to the cricothyroid membrane through which a trachaeostomy or tracheal tube can be inserted.[10] The patient can then be attached to a bag/valve device or a ventilator.

Cervical spine immobilisation

A cervical spine injury must be suspected in any patient with multi-system trauma, especially with an altered level of consciousness or blunt injury above the clavicles.[4] Care should be taken to keep the spine in alignment until:

- The patient is fully alert with a Glasgow Coma Scale of 15, AND
- A senior clinician has examined the spine, AND
- If necessary, x-rays have been taken and reported as normal.

Whilst in the ED, the patient should be immobilised by:

- Application of a correctly sized semi-rigid collar, and manual immobilisation, or
- Application of a correctly sized semi-rigid collar, head blocks and straps.

'A semi-rigid collar does not completely immobilise the spine, it is a flag that says; protect the neck, it might be injured'.[11] Whilst applying the collar and/or immobilisation the neck should be checked for wounds or signs of injury. The position of the trachea should be noted to ascertain if it is central or deviated, which may indicate thoracic injury.

If the immobilised patient needs to vomit, do one of two things:

Rapidly gather four people to carry out a log roll (Figure 2.4). The patient can then vomit whilst on their side. A fifth person should be available to assist and support the patient.

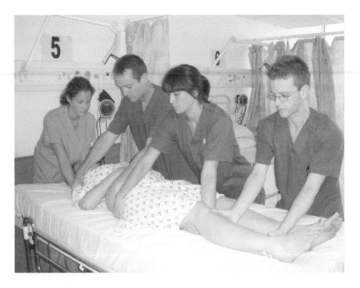

Fig. 2.4 Four-person log roll

OR

If four people are not available, tilt the bed or trolley head down. If the patient vomits, the vomitus will flow away from the face and head, away from the trolley. This is very unpleasant for the patient, however it minimises the risk of choking and aspiration. Remove the rigid suction catheter from the suction tubing and use the wide bore suction tubing to clear the secretions.

Breathing and ventilation

The body requires oxygen to produce cellular energy (aerobic metabolism). If there is a reduction in normal oxygen levels (hypoxia) due to traumatic injury then energy is produced without oxygen (anaerobic metabolism). This is an inefficient method of energy production and will result in the build up of lactate, with the patient eventually suffering from a metabolic acidosis.[12]

To minimise the risk of this, *all trauma patients need early supplemental oxygen.* In the self-ventilating patient this should be administered 15 L/min via a non-rebreathe mask with a reservoir bag. Using this method, an inspired oxygen concentration of approximately 85% can be achieved.[8] For the apnoeic patient or the patient struggling to breathe, assisted ventilation using a bag-valve-mask device, at 12–16 breaths per minute (adults) should be instigated, and expert help sought immediately.

To assess breathing and ventilation, a look, listen and feel approach should be adopted. Abnormal findings should be reported and acted on immediately.

Look

The chest should be fully exposed to allow for a comprehensive assessment. The chest is inspected for:

- Respiratory rate – tachypnoea (a high respiratory rate) may be due to hypoxia, hypovolaemia or pain
- Respiratory depth – shallow breathing may indicate increasing respiratory difficulty
- Respiratory effort – use of accessory muscles indicates that the patient is struggling to breath and will tire
- Symmetry of chest movements – injury such as fractures or a pneumothorax can cause asymmetry
- Wounds, abrasions, contusions – may indicate an underlying injury.

Oxygen saturation and CO_2 (if intubated) monitoring should be 'looked at' to assess ventilation. An arterial blood gas measurement (ABGs) may be necessary if hypoxia or hypoventilation is detected. Many seriously injured patients will suffer from inadequate organ perfusion and tissue oxygenation, therefore ABGs will accurately measure ventilation.

Listen

Listening to the patient's breathing during the assessment may reveal:

- Stridor (a crowing noise) which may indicate an airway obstruction
- Wheeze, especially following a burn injury, possibly indicating airway burns or inflammation.

Auscultation with a stethoscope is carried out to listen for:

- The presence of breath sounds in the anterior chest
- The presence of breath sounds in the axillae.

Feel

Each side of the chest wall should be gently examined, from clavicles to the rib borders, and the sternum for:

- Bony tenderness
- Crepitus (crunching).

The chest should be percussed by a trained clinician to elicit if there is air or blood trapped in the chest cavity (see Chapter 4, thoracic trauma)

Circulation and haemorrhage control

Haemorrhage is the main cause of early trauma deaths.[5]
   Common sites of haemorrhage include:

- The chest
- The abdomen
- The pelvis
- Long bones
- External haemorrhage from wounds/amputations.

Clinical examination, x-rays and FAST scanning (see Chapter 6, abdominal injuries) will be used to detect the site of bleeding. Expert help should be accessed promptly in order to arrest haemorrhage and prevent the patient deteriorating into irreversible hypovolaemic shock. Direct pressure should be applied to all external haemorrhage, and wounds should be checked beneath dressings to ensure that there isn't active bleeding.

Hypovolaemic shock

Case study 2.2 Compensation

A 27-year-old motorcyclist is involved in a collision with a tree at speed. He is thrown from his bike, landing on his front. After careful extrication at the scene he is immobilised and brought to the ED with high flow oxygen in situ.

A – airway is clear on arrival, the patient is talking
B – he is spontaneously breathing with a respiratory rate of 26
C – he is very anxious, has a pulse of 97 and a BP of 128/79
D – he is alert but anxious, GCS 15
E – he looks pale, with obvious bilateral femoral injuries.

30 minutes into his resuscitation his pulse is high at 110 however his BP remains at 125/80. He has not passed urine since the accident but is complaining of feeling 'dry'.

Despite his normal blood pressure, the team leader asks for 500 ml of intravenous fluids to be commenced, blood to be taken for group and cross matching and a urinary catheter to be inserted to monitor fluid balance. The student nurses watching the resuscitation question why he is deemed to be in hypovolaemic shock when his BP is within the normal range.

In the initial stages of haemorrhage compensatory mechanisms occur to help to maintain blood perfusion to the brain, heart and other vital organs. Compensation is caused by increased sympathetic activity and catecholamine (adrenaline and noradrenaline) release:[13,14]

- Catecholamines cause the heart rate to increase therefore the patient will be tachycardic.

• Systemic vasoconstriction helps to maintain the blood pressure, therefore the patient may appear to have a normal BP until a significant amount of blood loss has occurred.

Reduction in blood flow to the kidneys due to haemorrhage causes other compensatory mechanisms to occur. Antidiuretic hormone (ADH) together with aldosterone, reabsorbs sodium and water resulting in oliguria (reduced urine output). Angiotension II causes further vasoconstriction to help to maintain blood pressure within normal limits in the early stages of hypovolaemic shock.

Assessment of circulation

Assessment of the patient's circulatory status may reveal signs of hypovolaemic shock. Table 2.2 illustrates altered vital signs in the trauma patient and their significance.

For all trauma patients assessment of circulation should include:

• Heart rate
• Blood pressure
• Level of consciousness (mentation)

Table 2.2 Altered vital signs in response to haemorrhage

Heart rate	Tachycardia due to adrenaline and noradrenaline release *(tachycardia is an early sign!)* NB: Patients who are on beta blockers or patients who are very athletic will not appear to be tachycardic, although they may be hypovolaemic
Weak pulse	Due to reduced stroke volume
Altered mentation	Anxiety or confusion due to the reduction in brain perfusion
Capillary refill time	Delayed >2 seconds due to systemic vasoconstriction
Blood pressure	Normal or raised due to systemic vasoconstriction *(hypotension is a late sign!)*
Skin colour	Pale, cool peripheries due to systemic vasoconstriction. Sweating may be present due to catecholamine activity
Urine output	Reduced urine output and increased urine concentration due to ADH and aldosterone

- Capillary refill time
- Skin colour
- Urine output
- A 12 lead ECG for all patients over the age of 40 to detect concurrent cardiac problems.

Cardiac output monitoring is being used in some EDs. Ultrasound is used to measure the velocity and direction of the cardiac blood flow, accurately predicting cardiac output.

Cannulation and fluid resuscitation

Intravenous access should be obtained with two large cannulae. Blood should be taken for the following tests (however local guidelines should be adhered to):

- Full blood count
- Urea and electrolytes
- Group and save (or cross match if the patient needs a blood transfusion)
- Blood gases
- Blood clotting levels – many patients develop coagulopathy (clotting problems) caused by severe injury, therefore an early coagulation screen is important.[13]

Intravenous fluid therapy may be necessary if the patient is hypovolaemic. Isotonic crystalloid fluids are recommended such as 0.9% saline or Hartmann's solution.[5,15]

For many years the standard approach to the hypotensive trauma patient has been to infuse large volumes of intravenous fluid.[16] The aim was to restore and maintain a normal blood pressure, and was based on controlled animal experiments. This means that blood was withdrawn from the animal via a cannula until signs of hypovolaemic shock were present and then intravenous fluid was administered to replace the blood loss.[17]

However, contemporary fluid resuscitation is changing, as most traumatic haemorrhage is *uncontrolled* rather than

---

> **Box 2.4 Potentially harmful effects of traditional fluid replacement**
>
> - Increases blood pressure, which may dislodge early thrombi/clots
> - Cause a dilutional coagulopathy
> - Decrease oxygen delivery
> - Worsen metabolic acidosis
> - Cause hypothermia

controlled. Evidence from both human and animal studies now recommends a more cautious approach to fluid administration.[16,17]

The premise of *permissive hypotension* or *low volume fluid resuscitation* is that by restoring the blood pressure to 'normal' parameters, clots that may have formed will be dislodged by the fluid causing the patient to start to bleed (Box 2.4). Therefore, small volumes of fluid should be given (e.g. 250 ml boli in adults), allowing the vital organs to be perfused but reducing the risk of the problems seen in Box 2.4. If fluid is administered, the patient should be carefully assessed to see if they:

- Respond to the fluid and improve, or
- Respond to the fluid temporarily and then deteriorate again, or
- Do not respond to the fluid.

Temporary responders or non-responders are unstable, high risk patients. *Focus should be placed on finding the source of bleeding and accessing expert help to stop the haemorrhage early.*

Blood transfusion may be necessary for trauma patients with severe haemorrhage,[18] where the following may be prescribed to enhance oxygen delivery and assist with normal clotting:

- Packed red blood cells
- Fresh frozen plasma
- Cryoprecipitate.

Disability and dysfunction

Assessment of the level of consciousness should be carried out on all patients. Deterioration in conscious levels may be caused by:

- Hypoxia
- Hypovolaemia
- Head injury – raised intracranial pressure
- Medication of recreational drugs such as opiates
- Hypoglycaemia
- Hypothermia
- Alcohol ingestion.

A patient who has ingested alcohol or recreational drugs can be difficult to assess, and neurological symptoms may be masked. An intoxicated trauma patient's symptoms should never be dismissed as being caused by alcohol or drugs. All altered levels of consciousness should be attributed to injury until proven otherwise.

Assessment of consciousness can be carried out by using one of two methods: AVPU or the Glasgow Coma Scale.[8]

AVPU

Is the patient ALERT?
Is the patient responding to your VOICE?
Is the patient only responding to PAIN?
Is the patient UNRESPONSIVE?

If the patient is anything less than alert, further investigation should be carried out with the GCS.

Glasgow Coma Scale

The Glasgow Coma Scale is used to assess level of consciousness.[19] The patient's eye opening, verbal response and motor function are assessed and given a numerical rating between 3 (the worst score) and 15 (the best score). See Chapter 3 for further details.

If the patient has sustained a head injury and there is a risk of raised intracranial pressure, pupil size, equality and reaction should be assessed.

A blood sugar measurement should be taken to rule out hypoglycaemia.

Exposure and environmental control

The remainder of the patient's clothes should be removed to allow for a full examination, ensuring that the patient's dignity is maintained. The patient should not be allowed to become hypothermic, and should be covered whilst not being examined.[8]

All areas of the body, front and back, should be examined to ensure that potentially life-threatening injuries are not missed. This should include:

- Axillae
- Groin
- Back of head and neck
- Back of chest
- Lower back
- Buttocks.

A log roll will be necessary to allow the back examination, so that the spine is kept in alignment. This requires four people, with a fifth to conduct the examination. The correct position for a log roll is (Figure 2.4):

- Person 1 – holds the sides of the neck, keeping the head and neck still.
- Person 2 – places one hand on the patient's shoulder and one above the waist.
- Person 3 – places one hand on the patient's hip and one under the thigh.
- Person 4 – places one hand under the patient's knee and one under the ankle.

A clinician may perform a rectal examination to ensure that sphincter tone is intact (see Chapter 5) and whether there are signs of a pelvic fracture (see Chapter 7).

Analgesia

There is no excuse for leaving a trauma patient in pain.[20] Splinting of fractures should be carried out early and all patients in pain should be prescribed opiate analgesia, such as:

- Morphine 0.1 mg/kg IV or
- Ketamine 0.5–1 mg/kg IV.

These medications should be administered in small titrated amounts, e.g. 2–3 mg of morphine at a time, assessing pain following each dose. An antiemetic such as cyclizine or metochlopramide should be prescribed with the analgesia to avoid nausea and vomiting.

Tetanus

If there has been a breach in the patient's skin then there is a risk of tetanus infection. The bacteria *Clostridium tetanii* is found in the soil and animal faeces, and it enters the circulatory system through a wound. The effects of tetanus are generally controlled in Britain by an immunisation programme, however if acquired the disease can prove fatal.[21] Tetanus immunoglobulin should be reserved for patients with high risk wounds (those that have been in contact with animal faeces for example), who have never received primary immunisation.[22] See Table 2.3 for the Department of Health recommendations for tetanus immunisation.[23]

Diagnostic imaging

If chest or pelvic fractures are suspected, x-rays of these areas may be requested and carried out during the initial assessment phase. An x-ray of the cervical spine is usually necessary in blunt trauma to detect bony injury. However, in some hospitals, the cervical spine is imaged using a CT scan instead of an x-ray (see Chapter 5), especially if the head is to be scanned.

Table 2.3 Immunisation recommendations for clean and tetanus-prone wounds

Immunisation status	Clean wound	Tetanus-prone wound	Tetanus-prone wound
	Tetanus vaccine	**Tetanus vaccine**	**Human tetanus immunoglobulin**
Fully immunised, i.e. has received a total of five doses of vaccine at appropriate intervals	None required	None required	High risk wounds only
Primary immunisation complete, boosters incomplete but up to date	None required	None required	High risk wounds only
Primary immunisation incomplete or boosters not up to date	A reinforcing dose of tetanus vaccine and further doses as required to complete the recommended 5 doses	A reinforcing dose of tetanus vaccine and further doses as required to complete the recommended 5 doses	One dose of human tetanus immunoglobulin is required to be given in a different site
Not immunised or immunisation status not known or uncertain	An immediate dose of tetanus vaccine and then completion of a full five dose course	An immediate dose of tetanus vaccine and then completion of a full five dose course	One dose of human tetanus immunoglobulin is required to be given in a different site

SECONDARY SURVEY

Once the primary survey, or initial assessment, has been completed and the patient has not had to leave the ED for specialist input, a head to toe, back and front examination should be performed to ensure that injuries have not been missed. This should include assessment of:

- The head and scalp
- The face
- The neck
- The chest
- The abdomen
- The back
- Extremities
- Wounds.

Whilst the patient remains in the ED there should be close observation of vital signs and level of consciousness so that any deterioration in the patient's condition would lead to a reassessment of ABCDE.

If the patient is awake, or if relatives are present, past medical history can be obtained. This is most easily recounted using the AMPLE mnemonic:[2]

A Allergies
M Medication
P Past medical history
L Last food or drink
E Events relating to the history (e.g. chest pain whilst driving the car).

Documentation

Documentation of the initial assessment must be accurate and reflect the care and treatment that has been carried out. In many EDs a designated trauma booklet or sheet may be used to avoid fragmentation of notes.[2] See Chapter 13 for guidance on accurate documentation.

Property

It is also a nursing responsibility to record patient's property and valuables, and any interaction with the police, including handing over of forensic evidence (see Chapter 13).

Care of relatives and friends

In addition to caring for the trauma patient, consideration should be given to relatives or friends during the early stages of trauma care.[2] It will be a very anxiety provoking time for those close to the patient. All members of the ED team who come into contact with these people should be honest, sensitive and caring in their approach. A designated member of staff should be assigned to liaise with family members or close friends during the trauma resuscitation.[24] Opportunity to see the patient should be offered at an appropriate time during the resuscitation. Some departments operate a witnessed resuscitation policy where a close relative or friend may be present during the trauma assessment, supported by a member of ED staff.[2]

Transfer to definitive care

The patient may need to be transferred to definitive care, such as:

- Theatres
- Intensive care unit
- A high dependency unit
- A hospital ward or designated trauma ward.

Admission to definitive care requires clear communication and coordination to ensure appropriate, safe and timely transfer of the patient.[2] Prior to leaving the ED the following should be checked:

- Accurate patient ID bands
- Patients notes and x-rays (including the name of the person or team responsible for the patient care)

- Transfer oxygen, masks, suction, monitoring and resuscitation equipment
- Prescribed fluids and medication.

CONCLUSION

The trauma patient should be assessed and resuscitated in a timely manner to ensure that injuries are not missed. This may occur in the pre-hospital setting or the ED, by a small or large appropriately trained team. A systematic approach to the primary assessment, following A,B,C,D and E, will help to identify early life-threatening problems such as hypoxia or hypovolaemia. Specialist help should be summoned early to ensure that priorities such as timely diagnostic imaging and surgical intervention are available. In addition to patient assessment, consideration should be given to documentation, communication with relatives and liaison with definitive care.

KEY INFORMATION BOX

- Successful trauma teams need to be trained in both clinical care and human factors
- If the patient isn't talking, can they maintain their own airway?
- All trauma patients need high flow oxygen delivered by a non-rebreathe mask
- Tachycardia, tachypnoea and a reduced level of consciousness are all EARLY signs of hypovolaemic shock
- Compensatory mechanisms help to maintain the BP within normal limits in the early stages of hypovolaemic shock
- High volumes of intravenous fluids may be detrimental – find the bleeding and seek expert help early
- Trauma patients need adequate opiate analgesia.

REFERENCES

1. Davies G, Lockey D (2005) Prehospital care in trauma patients. In: Critical care focus 11: Trauma (Ed Galley H), 76–83. Blackwell Publishing, Oxford
2. Cole E, McGinley A (2005) A structured approach to caring for the trauma patient. In: Principles and practice

of trauma nursing (Ed O'Shea R), 37–60. Elsevier, Edinburgh

3. Cole E, Crichton N (2006) The culture of a trauma team in relation to human factors. Journal of Clinical Nursing 15:1257–1266

4. Findlay G, Martin IC, Carter S, Smith N, Weyman D, Mason M (2007) Trauma: who cares? A report on the National Confidential Enquiry into Patient Outcome and Death (NCEPOD), 10–14. NCEPOD, London

5. American College of Surgeons Committee on Trauma (2004) Initial assessment and management. In: Advanced trauma life support for doctors. Student course manual (7th edn), 11–32. American College of Surgeons, Chicago

6. Demetriades D, Berne TV (2004) Initial assessment and resuscitation of the injured patient. In: Assessment and management of trauma (Eds Demetriades D, Berne TV), 3–9. LAC & USC Healthcare Network, Los Angeles

7. Mikhail J (1999) The trauma triad of death: hypothermia, acidosis and coagulopathy. Advanced Practice in Acute Critical Care Issues 10:85–94

8. Greaves I, Porter KM, Ryan JM (Eds) (2001) Patient assessment. In: Trauma care manual, 18–32. Arnold, London

9. American College of Surgeons Committee on Trauma (2002) Airway and ventilatory management. In: Advanced trauma life support (7th edn), 41–52. American College of Surgeons, Chicago

10. Hodgetts T, Turner L (2006) Trauma rules 2 (2nd edn), 47. Blackwell Publishing, Oxford

11. Hodgetts T, Turner L (2006) Trauma rules 2 (2nd edn), 50–51. Blackwell Publishing, Oxford

12. Matthews W, Bentley P (2005) Applied biochemistry pertaining to the trauma patient. In: Principles and practice of trauma nursing (Ed O'Shea R), 119–128. Elsevier, Edinburgh

13. Bench S (2004) Clinical skills: assessing and treating shock: a nursing perspective. British Journal of Nursing 13:715–721

14. Brohi K, Singh J, Heron M, Coats T (2003) Acute traumatic coagulopathy. Journal of Trauma, Injury, Infection and Critical Care 54:1127–1130

15. Rizoli S (2002) Crystalloids and colloids in trauma resuscitation: a brief overview of the current debate. Journal of Trauma, Injury, Infection and Critical Care 54:S82–S88

16. Stern S (2001) Low volume fluid resuscitation for presumed haemorrhagic shock: helpful or harmful? Current Opinion in Critical Care 7:422–430

17. Revell M, Greaves I, Porter K (2003) Endpoints for fluid resuscitation in hemorrhagic shock. Journal of Trauma, Injury, Infection and Critical Care 54:S63–S67

18. Criddle L, Eldredge D, Walker J (2005) Variables predicting trauma patient survival following massive transfusion. Journal of Emergency Nursing 31:236–242

19. Teasdale G, Jennett B (1974) Assessment of coma and impaired consciousness. A practical scale. Lancet 2(7872): 81–84

20. Hodgetts T, Turner L (2006) Trauma rules 2 (2nd edn), 95–96. Blackwell Publishing, Oxford

21. Cassell O (2002) Death from tetanus after pre tibial laceration. BMJ 324:1442–1443

22. Rhee P, Nunley MK, Demetriades D, Velmahos G, Doucet JJ (2005) Tetanus and trauma: a review and recommendations. Journal of Trauma, Injury, Infection and Critical Care 58:1082–1088

23. Department of Health (2006) Immunisation against infectious disease – 'The Green Book': tetanus, chapter 30. http://www.dh.gov.uk/en/Policyandguidance/Health-andsocialcaretopics/Greenbook/DH_4097254

24. Cole E (2004) Assessment and management of the trauma patient. Nursing Standard 18(41):45–51

Head Injuries

3

Elaine Cole

INTRODUCTION

Head injuries are a common presentation to Emergency Departments (ED) and are a significant cause of morbidity and mortality. It is estimated that between 200 and 300 per 100,000 of the population in the UK are admitted to hospital each year with a head injury.[1] More than 50% of all major trauma cases sustain a severe head injury, resulting in 5000 fatalities per annum.[2] Severe head injuries most often result from falls (40%), violence (20%) and road traffic accidents (13%).[2] The key to successful assessment and management of patients with head injuries is to determine which of them has an underlying brain injury.

The aim of this chapter is to understand the principles of rapid assessment, resuscitation and stabilisation of the person with a head injury.

LEARNING OBJECTIVES

By the end of this chapter the reader will be able to:

❏ Identify the anatomical areas where traumatic head injuries occur
❏ Identify common head and brain injuries
❏ Define primary and secondary brain injury
❏ Understand factors that affect intracranial pressure and cerebral perfusion pressure
❏ Describe assessment and management priorities in relation to ABCDE.

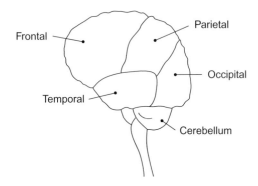

Fig. 3.1 Regions of the head and brain

ANATOMY

The head is divided up into four areas – frontal, temporal, parietal and occipital (Figure 3.1). Head injuries may involve one or a number of structures within these areas, including the scalp, bone, brain tissue and blood vessels.

Scalp

The scalp is made up of five layers and may be remembered using the mnemonic SCALP:

- Skin
- subCutaneous tissue
- galea Aponeurosis (a fibrous muscle layer)
- Loose areola tissue (beneath the galea where emissary veins are situated. These connecting veins drain blood from the sinuses in the dura to the central circulation)
- Periosteum.

Scalp wounds and haematomas confirm that there has been an injury to the head, and may indicate underlying bone or brain tissue damage. However, an intact scalp does not rule out a significant brain injury. Isolated scalp wounds are rarely life threatening, nevertheless they can be associated with significant bleeding, requiring careful exploration and closure.

Bone

Once the fontanelles have fused, the skull or cranium is a 'fixed box', which protects the brain. The facial bones provide a structure for the face. Fractures of the skull are described according to shape, site and displacement, and whether they are depressed or not.

Linear fractures

Linear fractures are usually caused by blunt trauma and consist of a line or crack in the bone. In the temporal region the bone is thin and closely associated with the middle meningeal artery.[3] A fracture in this region can tear the artery, which is a common cause of an extradural haematoma (discussed later).

Linear fractures may not necessarily need any treatment, however there is a risk of underlying brain injury. For this reason any patient in whom there is clinical suspicion of a skull fracture should have a CT scan.[3]

Depressed or compound fractures

Injury to the skull when bone is displaced inwards is known as a depressed skull fracture. The bone can be broken into a number of pieces (described as comminuted) and if there is an associated scalp wound present then the fracture is classified as being open or compound. Depressed fragments of bone can damage the underlying brain tissue, therefore an early neurosurgical referral should be made.[2] Compound skull fractures pose a risk of infection, therefore tetanus prophylaxis and antibiotics are required.

Base of skull fractures

The base of the skull is composed of five areas:

- Base of the orbit
- Sphenoid (part of the ethmoid bone)
- Temporal bone
- Occiput
- Cribriform plate.

Some clinical signs may indicate that a base of skull fracture is present.[2,3]

Frontal base of skull fractures may present with:

- Subconjunctival haemorrhage – the border of the clot on the sclera extends to back of the eyeball.
- Periorbital bruising or *racoon eyes* – this may indicate a base of skull fracture or it may indicate haemorrhage collected beneath the galea aponeurosis.
- Rhinorrhea – cerebrospinal fluid (CSF) leak from the nose (indicating a tear in the dura mater).

Mid base of skull fractures may present with:

- Otorrhea – CSF leak from the ear (indicating a tear in the dura mater).
- Haemotypanum – blood behind the tympanic membrane.
- Mastoid process bruising or *Battle's sign* (NB this will only develop after 4–6 hours in a supine patient).

Facial fractures

Fractures of the facial bones and underlying tissue injury are not generally life threatening unless they compromise the airway or cause severe haemorrhage.[4] However, facial fractures associated with head injuries are often caused by severe force, such as a head hitting the windscreen in a road traffic accident or assault to the head and face with a blunt object. Patients may present with obvious bleeding, facial swelling and facial deformity. Fractures of the middle third of the face can be broadly placed into one of three categories (Figure 3.2):

- Le Fort I – involving the maxilla
- Le Fort II – involving the maxilla and the nasal bones
- Le Fort III – involving the maxilla, the nasal bones and the zygomatic bones.

Le Fort III injuries are the most serious as they may result in airway compromise. Injuries which cause severe nasal bleeding may be managed by using nasal compression balloons (Epistats) or nasal packing.

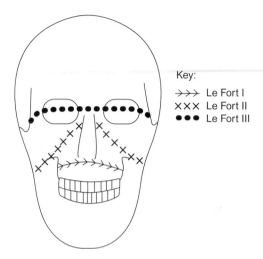

Key:
⟩⟩⟩ Le Fort I
✕✕✕ Le Fort II
●●● Le Fort III

Fig. 3.2 Le Fort fractures

Meninges

The meninges are situated between the inside of the skull and the brain (Figure 3.3).

The meninges consist of three layers:

- The dura mater – the outer fibrous membrane that lies close to the skull.
- The arachnoid layer – the soft cobweb-like structure beneath which cerebrospinal fluid (CSF) circulates.
- The pia mater – the soft membrane that is attached to the outer surface of the brain.

Brain

The brain is composed of the cerebrum (divided into two cerebral hemispheres), the cerebellum and the brainstem. Within the brainstem there is:

- The midbrain (containing the reticular activating system responsible for the awake state)

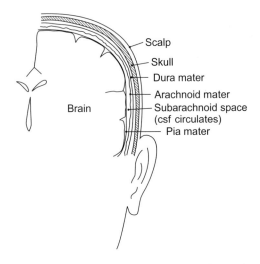

Fig. 3.3 Cross section of the head and brain including the meninges

- The pons and the medulla (which contains the cardiorespiratory control centres).

The tentorium is a fold of the dura mater that separates the cerebral hemispheres from the cerebellum and the brainstem.

PHYSIOLOGY

Primary and secondary brain injuries

Injuries to the brain can be described as primary or secondary.[2,5]

Primary injury occurs at the time of the incident and is irreversible. These injuries can be focal, affecting one area of the brain. These include:

- Contusions
- Haematomas
- Lacerations.

Injuries can be diffuse affecting the whole brain, including concussion and shearing injuries.

Secondary damage, which may be preventable or reversible, occurs at a later stage due to:

- Brain tissue hypoxia
- Oedematous brain tissue
- Systemic hypotension, causing the brain to be underperfused.

The main goal of treating head injuries is to recognise the primary injury and reduce or prevent the secondary brain injury.

In order to do this it is essential that intracranial pressure and cerebral perfusion pressure are understood.

Intracranial pressure

Three components are responsible for regulating intracranial pressure (ICP):[6]

$$\text{Volume of the brain} + \text{volume of CSF} + \text{volume of cerebral blood} = ICP$$

If one of the three components increases, such as the volume of the brain due to a haemorrhage, then there is a compensatory decrease in the other two components, allowing more space for the swollen brain:

- Vasoconstriction occurs reducing the volume of cerebral blood flow
- CSF production decreases and CSF gets displaced into the spinal subarachnoid space.

This process is called autoregulation, which helps to maintain the ICP within the normal range of 0–15 mmHg.

Autoregulation can only occur up to a point and once the ICP rises above 20 mmHg the compensatory mechanisms described above fail. Sustained ICP of >20 mmHg is associated with poor outcome for the head injured patient.[6]

In the severely head injured patient with a raised ICP, alteration of the cerebral blood vessels occurs. The cerebral vascular resistance increases causing the blood pressure to rise, to try to overcome the raised ICP. This hypertension associated with severe head injuries is known as *Cushing's response*[2] and is a late sign.

Cerebral perfusion pressure

The cerebral blood flow in the brain is approximately 700 ml/min.[7] This is maintained at a relatively constant rate by the constriction and dilation of the cerebral vessels. In order to ensure that the brain tissue is well oxygenated and perfused it is essential that cerebral perfusion pressure (CPP) is maintained within normal limits, 60–70 mmHg.

CPP is calculated thus:

$$\text{Mean arterial pressure (MAP)} + \text{ICP} = \text{CPP}$$

MAP is calculated by taking one-third of the difference between the systolic and diastolic blood pressure and adding it to the diastolic. See Box 3.1 for an example.

In an adult, the CPP should be maintained >70 mmHg and in young children >50 mmHg. A CPP of <50 mmHg is associated with ischaemic brain injury.

In a normotensive patient with no brain injury and a presumed normal ICP the CPP will be within normal limits. See Box 3.2 for an example.

However, in a traumatically injured patient who is hypovolaemic, hypotensive and has sustained a severe head injury

---

Box 3.1 Calculating mean arterial pressure

For a patient with a BP of 110/80 the MAP will be 90, calculated thus:

1/3 difference between the systolic and diastolic = 10
Therefore 10 + 80 (the diastolic) = MAP of 90

Box 3.2 Normal cerebral perfusion pressure

For a patient with a BP 110/80, the MAP will be 90

Subtract the ICP (normal range 0–15 mmHg)
90 (MAP) − 8 (ICP) = CPP 82 mmHg which is within normal
limits

Box 3.3 Altered cerebral perfusion pressure

For a patient with a BP 90/60, the MAP will be 70

Subtract the ICP (normal range 0–15 mmHg)
70 (MAP) − 20 ICP (raised due to an intracerebral injury) =
CPP 50 mmHg which suggests that the brain is at risk of
ischaemia

---

with a raised ICP, CPP may be compromised. See Box 3.3 for
an example.

Cerebral herniation

Case study 3.1 Cerebral herniation

A 21-year-old man has been involved in a fight. He was hit
on the head and face with a heavy object. Since arriving in
the ED his level of consciousness has decreased from a GCS
of 14 to a GCS of 9. On admission his pupils are equal and
reacting to light, size 4. The patient is intubated and GCS
observations continue to be recorded every 15 minutes,
whilst the patient awaits a CT scan. The nurse looking after
the patient notes that his right pupil is slightly larger than
his left and within 30 minutes the right pupil is size 7, fixed
and dilated whilst the left remains at size 4. The CT scan
shows a large extradural haematoma and the patient is
taken away for emergency surgery.

An expanding intracranial mass (such as a haematoma) or raising ICP can cause the brain to be forced downwards, known as herniation. During herniation, compression of the third cranial nerve – the ocular motor nerve, will cause a sluggish, dilating pupil on the affected side. Eventually if the swelling increases to such an extent that bilateral herniation has occurred, the patient will have bilateral fixed, dilated pupils. Progressively rising ICP causes further downward pressure of the brainstem known as *coning*.[1]

SPECIFIC BRAIN INJURIES

Concussion

Concussion is defined as a temporary loss of consciousness or cerebral disturbance with no long term neurological deficit following a head injury.[5] Some patients may complain of a headache, amnesia, and nausea or vomiting. Whilst there is no definitive treatment for concussion, a CT scan is warranted to rule out cerebral contusion. The patient can normally be discharged home following a normal CT with head injury instructions.

Contusion

Contusion is bruising of the brain tissue, often with associated swelling. This may be caused by the brain being shaken around in the skull (rapid acceleration – deceleration) or if the brain has been bruised by a bony prominence or skull fracture. Contusions are usually diagnosed on CT scan; however suspicion may be raised if the patient exhibits signs of prolonged loss of consciousness or reduced level of consciousness following the injury. Patients should be admitted to hospital to ensure that the contusion is not evolving into an intracerebral haematoma.[6] This is especially important for high risk patient groups such as those taking anti coagulants or with clotting disorders.

Traumatic axonal injury

Traumatic axonal injury usually results from a rapid acceleration–deceleration force, such as a high-speed road traffic accident. Stretching and shearing occurs causing swelling and injury to the axons within the brain tissue.[7] This can lead to permanent disability and is associated with high morbidity and mortality.

Extradural haematoma

An extradural haematoma is a bleed that occurs *outside* the dura mater beneath the skull (Figure 3.4). Classically it occurs due to an injury in the temporal region where branches of the middle meningeal artery are situated. Arterial injury causes bleeding, resulting in the dura being separated away from the skull. The expanding haematoma compresses the brain beneath it. Usually the bleed is rapid and the patient will quickly lose consciousness at the time of the injury occurring.

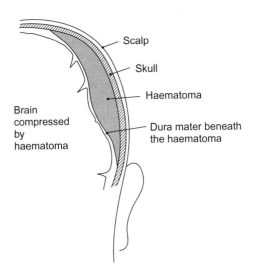

Fig. 3.4 Extradural haematoma

However, a proportion of patients will have a lucid period following the injury and then deteriorate swiftly into unconsciousness as the bleeding progresses.[1]

Following CT scan, patients with an extradural haematoma need emergency neurosurgery to evacuate the haematoma.

Subdural haematoma

This is the most common intracranial bleed associated with severe head injury and is associated with a worse outcome than for an extradural haematoma.[6] A haematoma forms *beneath* the dura mater as a result of injury to bridging veins (Figure 3.5).

A subdural haematoma can be acute or chronic. Acute injury usually manifests itself within the first few hours and can quickly evolve in size leading to reduced level of consciousness and coma. A CT scan will reveal the location of the haematoma and an urgent neurosurgical referral should be made for further management.

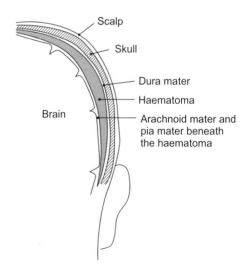

Scalp

Skull

Dura mater

Haematoma

Brain

Arachnoid mater and pia mater beneath the haematoma

Fig. 3.5 Subdural haematoma

Chronic subdural haematomas may appear days, weeks or months after the injury and they are common in small children and older patients. Venous in origin, bleeding is slow and there may be more space for the haematoma to build up due to a smaller or atrophied brain. This means that the signs and symptoms may be subtle and the patient deteriorates slowly. In the older patient, symptoms may be dismissed as confusion, dementia or falls. Once a chronic subdural haematoma has been confirmed on CT scan the patient should be referred to a neurosurgeon.

Intracerebral haematoma
An intracerebral haematoma is where bleeding has occurred deep within the brain tissue. These bleeds are often caused by severe force and may be associated with subdural haematoma. Following diagnosis on CT scan, an urgent neurosurgical referral is necessary. Patients with large intracerebral haematomas may need surgery, however smaller clots may be treated conservatively, with the patient closely observed for deterioration indicating an ongoing bleed or increasing intracranial pressure.

Penetrating injuries to the brain
Gunshot wounds to the brain are associated with very high mortality rates.[3] Other penetrating injuries can be sustained by objects such as knives or scissors being pushed through the skull with a great deal of force. If a patient presents with a penetrating object in situ, it must not be removed until the patient has had a CT scan and a senior surgeon is present.[3]

PRIMARY SURVEY ASSESSMENT AND RESUSCITATION
As part of the assessment process a number of important points from the history should be established which may give an indication of whether there has been an injury to the brain. These include:

- Mechanism of injury
- Whether or not there was a loss of consciousness or amnesia.

The conscious patient should be questioned about:

- The presence of a headache
- Nausea/vomiting
- Visual disturbances.

Airway with cervical spine control

As for all trauma patients, assessment of the airway with simultaneous cervical spine control is the first priority for the head injured patient. Any patient with a head or facial injury must be expected to have a cervical spine injury until proven otherwise by a senior clinician. There is a 5% association of cervical spine injury with severe head injury.[1]

Patients with a suspected base of skull fracture should not have a nasopharyngeal airway inserted because of the risk of passing the airway into brain tissue.

Early tracheal intubation is indicated for the head injured patient with a GCS < 9.[2] Patients with severe facial injuries that cannot maintain a patent airway due to bleeding, swelling or deformity, should be intubated early. Severe damage to the face and upper airway may mean that a surgical airway (as described in Chapter 2) is the most expedient method of securing a patent airway.

Breathing and ventilation

The brain needs to be adequately oxygenated in order to function normally. A head injured patient does not tolerate hypoxia well and a small decrease in oxygen levels reaching the brain can result in a reduced level of consciousness. *Therefore all head injured patients need 15 L/min high flow oxygen via a non-rebreathing mask.*

The assessment of breathing and ventilation is vitally important for the head injured patient. There is a direct relationship between the patient's carbon dioxide level ($PaCO_2$) and the diameter of their cerebral vessels.[2] High levels of $PaCO_2$, known as hypercarbia, cause cerebral vasodilation, which allows more blood flow to the brain. *This in turn will cause an increase in intracranial pressure.* Therefore, patients who cannot adequately self ventilate should be electively intubated and ventilated to control the breathing. It is recommended that the $PaCO_2$ levels should be maintained at 4–4.5 kPa/30–35 mmHg.

Hyperventilation is sometimes considered for patients with high levels of $PaCO_2$ under the direction of a senior clinician. Hyperventilation acts by 'blowing off' or reducing $PaCO_2$ and causing cerebral vasoconstriction. The $PaCO_2$ level should not be allowed to fall lower than 3.5 kPa/25 mmHg due to the risk of causing severe cerebral vasoconstriction with resulting ischaemia.[6,8]

Regular monitoring of the following is essential to ensure that ventilation is effective:

- Respiratory rate
- Respiratory depth
- Chest movements
- Oxygen saturations
- CO_2 trace (if the patient is intubated).

Circulation and haemorrhage control

It is essential to maintain blood flow to the brain. Hypotension can have devastating effects on cerebral blood flow and the ability to maintain CPP.[8] Hypotension with a systolic BP of 90 or less for the adult head injured patient doubles the risk of mortality.[5] Therefore, isotonic IV fluids such as normal saline should be given to maintain the BP.

Contemporary practice suggests that hypertonic saline (HTS) may be preferable for hypotensive patients with head injuries as the increased plasma osmolality causes water to move from the brain tissue into the intravascular space (thus reducing ICP). There is insufficient evidence to definitively recommend the use of HTS at the present time,[9] however some pre-hospital providers are administering HTS to head injured patients with positive effects.[10]

Case study 3.2 Re-assessment of the deteriorating patient

A 55-year-old cyclist is thrown from her bicycle following a collision with a van. On arrival to the ED she has a wound on her forehead, a swollen and deformed right leg and looks pale. Her GCS is 13 (her eyes are closed and she is confused), her pulse is 97 and her BP is 118/74.

Her primary survey assessment reveals that she needs a CT scan due to the head injury and that she has a fractured right tibia and fibula. All other x-rays and FAST scan are negative. Following her CT scan, which showed a small subdural haematoma, the patient is intubated and referred to neurosurgery. Her vital signs deteriorate with a pulse of 123 and a BP of 96/50.

The nurse caring for the patient speaks to the trauma team leader about the patient's deterioration and a second FAST scan of the abdomen is performed. This shows free fluid around the liver, and a surgeon is immediately called for.

Closed head injuries alone do not cause hypotension. If the patient is exhibiting signs of hypotension or shock this will *usually* be due to haemorrhage. In overwhelming head injuries, hypotension may present at a late stage, due to brainstem damage and may be a terminal sign.

Disability and dysfunction

The patient's level of consciousness should be formally assessed using the Glasgow Coma Scale (GCS) (Table 3.1). By adding together:

- The eye opening
- The best verbal response
- The best motor (movement) response.

Table 3.1 The Glasgow Coma Scale

Assessment	Score
Eye opening	
• Spontaneous	4
• To speech	3
• To pain	2
• No response	1
Verbal response	
• Orientated	5
• Confused conversation	4
• Inappropriate words	3
• Incomprehensible sounds	2
• No response	1
Best motor response	
• Obeys commands	6
• Localises pain	5
• Withdraws/flexes to pain	4
• Abnormal flexion	3
• Extension	2
• No response	1

A total score out of 15 can be established. If available, this score should be compared to a GCS measurement taken at the scene of the injury, to detect if there has been a neurological deterioration.

The GCS can be subjective and therefore a standard set of questions should be used to elicit if the patient is confused or using inappropriate words. If the patient is intubated and unable to verbally respond the number should be substituted with the letter T. When assessing motor function, limb injuries should be taken into account when asking the patient to move. If a painful stimulus has to be used to elicit a motor response, a central rather than peripheral site should be chosen, such as a trapezius pinch (the muscle between the shoulder and the neck) or a sternal rub.

The GCS is often used to help define the severity of traumatic brain injury:[6]

- Minor injuries are generally defined as those associated with a GCS score of 13–15.
- Moderate injuries are those associated with a GCS score of 9–12.
- Severe injuries are defined as those with a GCS score of 8 or less.

These definitions are not rigid and should be considered as a general guide to the level of injury in conjunction with history, examination and findings.[11]

Patients who have consumed alcohol or drugs prior to the head injury can be very difficult to assess. It should never be assumed that an altered level of consciousness is due to intoxication, and underlying brain injury must be ruled out.

A blood sugar measurement should be performed to ensure that the patient is not hypo- or hyperglycaemic.

Pupil size and reaction
Pupils should be assessed for size and reaction to light:

- Swollen, bruised eyelids should be carefully opened to see the pupil beneath. A closed eye due to a periorbital haematoma may be hiding a dilating pupil beneath the lid.
- A dilated pupil associated with a head injury could be indicative of pressure on the ocular motor nerve tract.
- 1 mm size difference is considered significant of injury.[6]

Altered pupil size and reaction is a later sign than reduction in level of consciousness However, if the patient has been paralysed, sedated and intubated, a dilated pupil may be the first sign of increasing ICP.[1] In a well, fully alert patient with a GCS of 15 who has unequal pupils, this may be due to an ophthalmic problem or previous eye surgery.

Assessment of the head
The ears and the nose should be checked for bleeding or a CSF leak, indicating a possible base of skull fracture. A high glucose measurement in the leaked fluid will determine if CSF is

present. Alternatively the halo test can be used, where a drop of the leaked fluid is placed in a white sheet (or blotting paper if available). Blood will stay in the centre of the drop and a clear ring of CSF will spread concentrically around it.

The scalp should be examined for wounds or contusions that may be indicative of an underlying injury. It is important to stop profuse bleeding from scalp wounds, especially in children and patients with a clotting disorder or on anticoagulants.

Exposure and environmental control

The patient should be fully undressed to allow for a thorough top to toe examination. If not already performed, a log roll should be carried out to allow an examination of the back of the head to ensure that no injuries are missed.

Severely head injured patients are at risk of developing hyperthermia due to damage to the hypothalamus.[1,12] Whilst this generally manifests itself once the patient is in the intensive care setting, pyrexia following head trauma is associated with worsened neurological outcome and should be noted in the ED. There is ongoing research investigating the possibilities of brain cooling but keeping the body temperature normal. This is not yet a concept that has been adopted for brain injured patients in the ED.

CT SCANNING FOR THE HEAD INJURED PATIENT

The primary investigation of choice for the detection of brain injuries is Computerised Tomography scanning (CT).[11] National guidance was published in 2003 suggesting that early CT scanning, rather than admission and observation for neurological deterioration, will reduce the time taken to detect life-threatening complications.[11] Any patient who presents with the following should have an urgent CT scan as part of the ED assessment process:[11]

- GCS less than 13 at any point since the injury
- GCS equal to 13 or 14 at 2 hours after the injury
- Suspected open or depressed skull fracture

- Any sign of basal skull fracture
- Post-traumatic seizure
- Focal neurological deficit
- More than one episode of vomiting
- Amnesia for greater than 30 minutes of events before the injury. The assessment of amnesia is unlikely to be possible in children aged under 5 years.

Other groups that should also be considered for an urgent CT scan are those who are intoxicated, patients over the age of 65, patients taking anticoagulants or those with altered clotting mechanisms.

The care of all patients with acute head injuries and an abnormal CT scan should be discussed with a neurosurgeon. Regardless of imaging, other reasons for discussing a patient's care with a neurosurgeon include:[11]

- Persisting coma (GCS less than or equal to 8) after initial resuscitation
- Unexplained confusion which persists for more than 4 hours
- A seizure without full recovery
- Definite or suspected penetrating injury
- A cerebrospinal fluid leak
- A depressed skull fracture.

TRANSFER PROTOCOLS

Transfer can be a time of great danger for the head injured patient. Moving patients from the emergency department in one hospital to a tertiary neurosurgical centre is a high risk procedure, which requires careful planning and management.[11] There should be a designated consultant in both the referring and the receiving hospitals who communicate to establish arrangements for the transfer of the patient. A doctor with at least two years' experience and training in anaesthesia and an appropriately skilled assistant should accompany the patient in the ambulance.[11] It is recommended that patients with a GCS of 8 or less must be intubated and ventilated prior to transfer. Other indications for intubation and ventilation include:[11]

- Hypoxia – PaO_2 of < 13 kPa on high flow oxygen
- Hypercarbia – $PaCO_2$ of > 6 kPa
- Significantly deteriorating conscious level
- Facial fractures/copious facial bleeding
- Seizures.

CONCLUSION

Initial assessment and management of the head injured patient should be centred on recognising primary injury and preventing secondary damage. Hypoxia, hypercapnia and hypotension should be prevented to optimise the patient outcome. Ongoing assessment of the GCS, early CT scanning and early involvement of a neurosurgeon should be key components of the patient's care.

KEY INFORMATION BOX

- A reduced level of consciousness is a significant indicator of brain injury
- The brain needs oxygen early
- Closed head injuries do not usually cause hypotension and tachycardia – is the patient bleeding somewhere?
- Allowing the patient to become hypotensive following a brain injury will be detrimental to CPP and cerebral blood flow
- An altered level of consciousness should never be attributed to alcohol or drugs until a head injury has been ruled out
- Prompt CT scanning is essential to diagnose brain injuries
- Transfer of a head injured patient is a high risk procedure and needs careful planning and preparation.

REFERENCES

1. Maartens N, Lethbridge G (2005) Head and neck trauma. In: Principles and practice of trauma nursing (Ed O'Shea R), 333–362. Elsevier, Edinburgh
2. Greaves I, Porter KM, Ryan JM (Eds) (2001) Head injuries. In: Trauma care manual, 99–114. Arnold, London

3. Marion DW (2002) Head injury. In: The trauma manual (2nd edn) (Eds Peitzman AB, Rhodes M, Schwab CW, Yealy DM, Fabian TC), 132–139. Lippincott, Williams & Wilkins, Philadelphia

4. Parkins DRJ (2005) Maxillofacial trauma. In: Principles and practice of trauma nursing (Ed O'Shea R), 457–468. Elsevier, Edinburgh

5. March K (2003) Head and neck trauma. In: Trauma nursing secrets (Ed Sauderson Cohen S), 61–75. Hanley & Belfus, Philadelphia

6. American College of Surgeons Committee on Trauma (2004) Head trauma. In: Advanced trauma life support for doctors. Student course manual (7th edn), 151–167. American College of Surgeons, Chicago

7. Gaetz M (2004) The neurophysiology of brain injury. Clinical Neurophysiology 115:4–18

8. Trauma.org (2000) Neurotrauma. Acute management of traumatic brain injury. http://www.trauma.org/neuro/acutemanagement.html 5.1

9. Jackson R, Butler J (2004) Best evidence topic report: hypertonic and isotonic saline in hypotensive patients with severe head injury. Emergency Medical Journal 21:80–81

10. Cooper DJ, Myles PS, McDermott FT, Murray LJ, Laidlaw J, Cooper G, Tremayne AB, Bernard SS, Posnford J (2004) Prehospital hypertonic saline resuscitation of patients with hypotension and severe traumatic brain injury: a randomised controlled trial. JAMA 291:1350–1357

11. National Institute for Health and Clinical Excellence (2007) Head injury. Triage, assessment, investigation and early management of head injury in infants, children and adults. Clinical guideline 56. http://www.nice.org.uk/nicemedia/pdf/word/CG56NICEguidelineword.doc

12. Andrews P (2005) Rationale for direct brain cooling after head injury. In: Critical care focus 11: Trauma (Ed Galley H), 52–62. Blackwell Publishing, Oxford

Thoracic Trauma

4

Elaine Cole

Severe injuries to the chest are common, accounting for 25% of all trauma deaths.[1] Thoracic injury, involving the lungs, heart, major vessels or bony structures, can be caused by blunt and penetrating trauma. Some thoracic injuries will cause immediate death, such as a traumatic aortic dissection. Other life-threatening thoracic injuries including airway obstruction, pnuemothoraces, major haemorrhage and cardiac tamponade need timely assessment and intervention.[2] Recognition of thoracic injury is focused on careful assessment, clinical examination and diagnostic imaging. Moreover, prompt life saving treatment of thoracic injuries involves airway management, delivery of oxygen, ensuring adequate ventilation, underwater seal chest drainage and haemorrhage control.[3,4]

The aim of this chapter is to understand the principles of rapid assessment, resuscitation and stabilisation of the person with a thoracic injury.

LEARNING OBJECTIVES

By the end of this chapter the reader will be able to:

❏ Describe the anatomy of the chest
❏ Understand common mechanisms of thoracic injury
❏ Identify major thoracic injuries
❏ Describe assessment and management priorities in relation to ABCDE
❏ Identify when a thoracotomy may be carried out in the emergency department (ED).

ANATOMY OF THE CHEST

Due to their close proximity, injury to the chest can involve many of the structures within the thorax. Figure 4.1 illustrates the structures located within the thorax.

These structures can be categorised into those that are situated in the thoracic cage and those in the thoracic cavity.[3]

The thoracic cage contains:

- 12 pairs of ribs attached to the thoracic spine posteriorly (at the back)
- The sternum (or breastbone) where ribs 1–7 attach anteriorly (at the front)
- The scapulae (or shoulder blades)
- Intercostal muscles which are located above and below each rib assisting with ventilation.

The thoracic cavity contains:

- The lower airways including trachea, right and left bronchi, bronchioles and alveoli

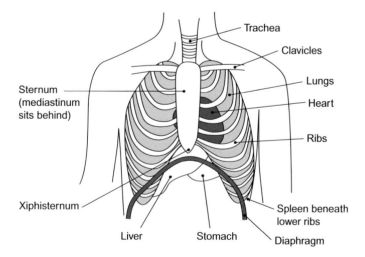

Fig. 4.1 Structures within the thorax

- The left and right lungs
- The great vessels such as the thoracic aorta, pulmonary arteries and pulmonary veins, inferior and superior vena cavae
- The mediastinum (the division between the two lungs which contains the heart, the trachea and the oesophagus)
- The heart.

The diaphragm, a large dome shaped muscle, separates the thorax from the abdomen.

The lungs
The right lung is divided into three lobes, upper, middle and lower, and the left lung is divided into two lobes, upper and lower. Covering each of the lungs are the pleura:

- The visceral layer of the pleura is the inner layer that lines the outer surface of the lungs
- The parietal layer of the pleura is the outer layer that lines the chest wall.

Between the layers of the pleura is a *potential space*. In normal respiration the pleura glide over each other, moistened by serous fluid. Following traumatic injury there is a risk that air or blood can enter the potential space causing the underlying lung to collapse (Figure 4.2).

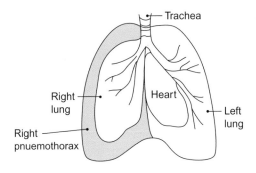

Fig. 4.2 Right pneumothorax

The heart

The heart is situated between the lungs, predominantly on the left side of the chest. The heart has three layers:

- The pericardium – outer layer
- The myocardium – middle layer
- The endocardium – inner layer.

The pericardium is a strong fibrous sac that is further subdivided into two layers:

- The inner visceral pericardium
- The outer parietal pericardium.

Traumatic injury can cause bleeding between the visceral and parietal pericardial layers, known as a cardiac tamponade, which compromises the contractions of the heart.

MECHANISM OF THORACIC INJURY

Blunt trauma

Blunt thoracic trauma can cause injury to any of the structures within the thoracic cage and thoracic cavity. The main mechanisms of injury caused by blunt trauma are:[3]

- Rapid deceleration
- Direct impact
- Compression.

Rapid deceleration

Trauma involving high speed, such as a road traffic accident (RTA) or fall from a height, may cause rapid deceleration injuries. The body gains momentum as the speed increases, then the body stops suddenly, e.g. hitting the ground following a fall, or hitting another vehicle at speed. The stabilising portion of the organ or vessel stops before the organ or vessel, causing a shearing or tearing injury,[5] which may result in haemorrhage.

Direct impact

Heavy or immovable objects impacting with the chest, such as a steering wheel or seat belt, cause direct impact injuries. Fractures of the bony rib cage and sternum may result, potentially injuring the underlying structures such as the lungs or heart.[3]

Compression

Crush injury to the chest can cause the structures within to be compressed and damaged. This can be due to an external crushing force such as a heavy vehicle or a collapsing wall. Alternatively internal crush injury can occur during rapid deceleration. Here, the chest organs are compressed from behind by the posterior chest wall and vertebral column, which continue to move forward after the anterior chest wall has come to a stop.[5]

Penetrating trauma

Thoracic injury may be caused by any object that penetrates the chest wall.[3] The penetrating object causes a chest wound and potentially injures the underlying structures.

Penetrating injury to the chest may be caused by:

- Guns
- Knifes
- Other sharp objects such as broken glass, pens, tools
- Impalement onto a fence or post
- Flying debris from a bomb blast or explosion.

All penetrating chest wounds should be explored by a senior clinician. Seemingly innocuous wounds may not reflect underlying damage. For example, a small, clean stab wound to the left axilla (armpit) may appear to be insignificant, however the knife blade may have penetrated the pericardium causing cardiac tamponade. Similarly a gunshot wound may appear to be small, however a bullet can travel on entering the body causing damage to thoracic organs and vessels.

A penetrating object to the chest wall that is still in situ should not be removed until the patient is in an operating theatre with a surgeon present, ready to operate.[3] The rationale for leaving the object in situ is that it may be compressing or tamponading vessels, which could start to bleed uncontrollably if the object is removed. This could prove catastrophic in an uncontrolled environment.

SPECIFIC THORACIC INJURIES

Major thoracic injuries can be divided into those that are immediately life threatening and those that are life threatening but are less obvious and often difficult to diagnose. The two groups of injuries have been described as the *Lethal six* and the *Hidden six*.[2] Table 4.1 shows the two groups.

The lethal six

Airway obstruction

If the airway is obstructed and not promptly opened then death will occur within minutes. Injury to the upper chest can affect the airway. A bone fragment from a fracture or a penetrating object may injure the larynx or upper trachea. Blunt trauma can cause haemorrhage or swelling in the airway, resulting in an obstruction.

Signs and symptoms suggestive of an airway obstruction:

- An unconscious patient with no air coming from the mouth and nose

Table 4.1 Major thoracic injuries

The lethal six	The hidden six
Airway obstruction	Traumatic aortic disruption
Massive haemothorax	Tracheobronchial tree injury
Tension pneumothorax	Oesophageal perforation
Open pneumothorax	Myocardial contusion
Cardiac tamponade	Pulmonary contusion
Flail chest	Diaphragmatic tear or rupture

- Noises – stridor, grunting, snoring
- Hoarseness or vocal changes in the conscious patient
- Obvious swelling, bleeding or bruising to the neck, clavicles or upper sternum.

Immediate treatment:

- Systematic airway opening manoeuvres as described in Chapter 2
- Endotracheal intubation performed by a senior clinician to secure a definitive airway.

Massive haemothorax

A massive haemothorax can be caused by blunt or penetrating trauma.[1,2] Injury to the lung tissue, pulmonary vessels and intercostal vessels can result in massive haemorrhage. Blood rapidly accumulates in the lung causing hypoxia and hypovolaemia.

A haemothorax is described as a massive haemothorax in the presence of >1500 ml blood loss in the chest drain or 200 ml per hour (3 mg/kg/hr).[1,2,4] On a chest x-ray the lung field may appear to be completely white. A smaller haemothorax may not show on a supine chest x-ray (where the patient is lying flat) and this will be detected by considering signs and symptoms, and clinical examination.

Signs and symptoms suggestive of a massive haemothorax:

- Shocked patient – altered level of consciousness, tachycardic, tachypnoeic, hypotensive
- Pallor
- Abrasions, wounds, injury to the affected side
- Asymmetrical breathing
- Reduced breath sounds on the affected side
- Hyporesonance (or dullness) to percussion on the affected side
- Ongoing blood loss in the chest drain bottle (as described above).

Immediate treatment:

- High flow oxygen
- Intravenous access established and blood taken for group and cross matching
- Chest tube insertion (tube thoracostomy) and underwater seal chest drainage (Box 4.1, Figure 4.3).

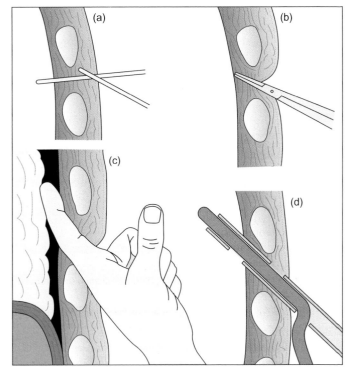

Fig. 4.3 Chest drain insertion. (Reproduced with permission from Hodgetts T, Turner L (2006) Trauma rules 2 (2nd edn), figure 54.1. Blackwell Publishing, Oxford)

Box 4.1 Tube thoracostomy and underwater seal drainage

- Reassure the patient and briefly explain the procedure
- The chest tube will be inserted in the 4th or 5th intercostal space, slightly anterior to the mid-axilliary line, therefore the patient's arm may need to be raised and supported
- Local anaesthetic such as lidocaine (lignocaine) 1% should be available
- Equipment: Chest drain insertion sterile set:
  - Scalpel
  - Sterile chest tube (size 32 fr or larger for an adult)
  - Underwater seal drainage system and bottle
  - Sterile water to add to the bottle up to the fill line
  - Large suture such as a hand held needle
  - Dressing if required (as per local policy)
- On the affected side, the clinician will anaesthetise the area, make an incision, dissect through to the pleura and then insert the tube
- Attach the prepared underwater seal drainage system
- The tube will be sutured into place and covered as per local policy
- Note if any blood drains, report the amount to the clinician in charge of the patient's care
- Observe for swinging or misting of the drainage tube, indicating that the lung is re-inflating
- Check the vital signs and pulse oximetry
- A chest x-ray should be performed to ensure correct tube placement

Thoracic suction may be applied to the chest drain bottle. This is normally indicated for a large haemothorax to remove the blood from the lung, allowing for improved ventilation or when a large air leak is present

The underwater seal system and bottle should always be kept below the level of the patient's chest. Do not clamp the chest drain except for during bottle change. Clamping increases the risk of causing a tension pneumothorax!

Tension pneumothorax

Caused by blunt or penetrating trauma, a tension pneumothorax develops when a 'one way valve' or flap occurs in the lung lining or chest wall.[4] On inhalation, the valve or flap opens and air enters the pleural space. On exhalation, the valve or flap closes so that the air cannot escape from the pleural space. The next breath allows more air in, again unable to escape. Air accumulates under pressure (*or tension*) within the pleural space causing the lung beneath to collapse. If the trapped air is not released, the tension will continue to build. This results in decreased venous return to the heart, and reduction in cardiac output. It may also cause a collapse of the unaffected lung and mediastinal deviation.

Signs and symptoms suggestive of a tension pneumothorax:

- An anxious, agitated patient
- Respiratory distress
- Tachycardia (possibly due to concurrent haemorrhage)
- Asymmetrical breathing – the chest may appear to be over-inflated on the affected side
- Absent breath sounds on the affected side
- Hyperresonance (high pitched sounds) on percussion of the affected side
- Distended neck veins (if not bleeding elsewhere)
- Possible deviated trachea away from the affected side (although this is an inconsistent sign).[6]

Immediate treatment:

- High flow oxygen (if the patient will tolerate this)
- *Immediate* chest x-ray to confirm the diagnosis
- Needle decompression of the affected lung (Box 4.2), converting a tension pneumothorax to a simple pneumothorax
- Chest tube insertion (tube thoracostomy) and underwater seal chest drainage.

Box 4.2 Needle decompression of a tension pneumothorax

- Reassure the patient and explain the procedure
- Local anaesthetic such as lidocaine (lignocaine) may be used however as this is a life saving procedure there may not be time
- Equipment: large bore cannula (14 or 16 gauge) and tape
- On the affected side, the clinician will insert the cannula into the 2nd intercostal space, mid-clavicular line, over the top of the 3rd rib
- The needle and cap will be removed – a hiss of air may be heard
- The cannula should be left in situ and taped securely

Open pneumothorax

Penetrating injury to the chest may result in an opening that goes from the external chest wall through to the lung. An open pneumothorax occurs when the wound remains open and the lung beneath collapses. If the wound is bigger than two-thirds of the diameter of the trachea (>3 cm in diameter) then air will preferentially be sucked in through the opening with each breath.[1,2,4] This is sometimes described as a *sucking chest wound*. Effective ventilation and gaseous exchange are impaired and the patient will become hypoxic.

Signs and symptoms suggestive of an open pneumothorax:

- Wound or opening on chest wall
- Respiratory distress
- Tachycardia, tachypnoea
- Patient anxiety or agitation
- Asymmetrical breathing
- Reduced breath sounds on the affected side
- Hyperresonance on percussion of the affected side.

Immediate treatment:

- High flow oxygen
- Placement of a dressing over the wound ONLY TAPED DOWN ON THREE SIDES – this prevents air entering the pleural space on inhalation and allows air to escape on exhalation[4]
- Chest tube insertion (tube thoracostomy) and underwater seal chest drainage (placed away from the wound).

Cardiac tamponade

Case study 4.1 Penetrating chest injury

A 17-year-old male is brought to the ED by friends. He has been involved in a fight outside of college and says that he has been stabbed. There is a gaping wound to his right cheek and both of his hands are bleeding. He is taken directly to the resuscitation room where high flow oxygen is applied, he is connected to a cardiac monitor and the trauma team are requested, his initial vital signs are:

RR 23, HR 111, BP 105/74

Intravenous access is secured and trauma bloods are sent to the lab. There are a number of scratches to his anterior chest, a large wound on his right hand and a smaller wound on his left hand. The patient is verbally aggressive, shouting and swearing. He is calling out for painkillers. 10 mg morphine IV is prescribed. Following administration of this his blood pressure drops to 88/56 and the patient is laid flat. An immediate FAST scan is requested which shows an effusion in his pericardium – with a diagnosis of cardiac tamponade. On further examination of his back a small stab wound is noted beneath his left scapula. A cardiothoracic surgeon is fast bleeped and the patient is taken to theatre for emergency surgery.

Penetrating trauma, e.g. a stab wound to the upper chest, is a common cause of cardiac tamponade. However severe blunt force may damage the heart and great vessels causing bleeding into the pericardium.[1] The fibrous pericardium fills with blood, restricting cardiac filling and contractions. Only a relatively small amount of bleeding is needed to compromise cardiac activity, such as 75–100 ml of blood.[2] Pericardiocentesis – inserting a needle into the pericardium to drain blood and therefore relieve cardiac compromise – is a blind technique that should only be used in peri-arrest situations. The technique may fail due to blood having clotted in the pericardium. An ultrasound or echo scan of the heart followed by surgery is recommended as optimal treatment.[6]

Signs and symptoms suggestive of a cardiac tamponade:

- A restless, anxious patient
- Shock – altered level of consciousness, tachycardia, hypotension without any areas of bleeding
- Pulsus paradoxus – a decrease of the systolic blood pressure by 10 mmHg on inspiration
- 'Beck's Triad' – hypotension, distended neck veins and muffled or distant heart sounds, however these are only present in a small percentage of patients and are difficult to assess in a noisy ED
- Raised CVP
- Cardiopulmonary arrest following thoracic trauma.

Immediate treatment:

- High flow oxygen
- Establish intravenous access
- ECG and cardiac monitoring
- FAST scan to look for pericardial fluid (see Chapter 6 for further details)
- Immediate referral to a cardiothoracic surgeon for possible operative management.

Flail chest

Blunt trauma, specifically direct impact and compression forces, are common causes of a fail chest. A segment of the bony rib cage is injured, often anteriorly (at the front) or laterally (at the side), causing a loss of continuity with the rest of the ribs. Classically a flail chest is defined as fractures of two or more ribs in two or more places.[1,4] The chest moves paradoxically, i.e. a segment of fractured ribs moves forward during inspiration whilst the rest of the bony cage moves backwards, and then vice versa on expiration. Hypoxia develops as the mobile flail segment injures the underlying lung tissue potentially causing pulmonary contusion.[4] If the patient is conscious and in pain, there may be a reluctance to breathe deeply causing hypoxia due to poor ventilation.

Signs and symptoms suggestive of a flail chest:

- Abnormal chest movements on the affected side (may not be seen if the patient is ventilated)
- Respiratory distress
- Use of accessory muscles
- Poor oxygen saturations
- Chest pain
- Bony crepitus (crunching) on palpation.

Immediate treatment:

- High flow oxygen
- Analgesia – intravenous morphine or regional analgesia such as an epidural or intercostal nerve block (no associated respiratory depression)
- Close monitoring of respiratory effort, oxygen saturations and arterial blood gases – the patient may need to be intubated and ventilated.

Fractures of the sternum, scapulae or first ribs are of particular significance. These bones require a great deal of force to cause an injury. If these fractures are diagnosed, senior help should be sought urgently to rule out underlying lung, great vessel or tracheobronchial injury.

The hidden six

Traumatic aortic disruption

A tear in the wall of the aorta is usually caused by rapid deceleration such as a high speed RTA, fall from a height or ejection from a vehicle. Many people with a traumatic aortic disruption (TDA) will die at the scene of the incident.[1,2] Of those that survive, the risk of aortic rupture is high. The aorta has three layers and the outer layer, the adventitia, is often the only thing that is containing the haematoma caused by the tear. If pressure is placed on the adventitia, by raising the patient's blood pressure, this layer can rupture causing major haemorrhage and death.

Signs and symptoms suggestive of a TDA:

- There may not be any obvious signs or symptoms, suspicion may come from the mechanism of injury
- Other injuries suggesting a large amount of blunt force such as a fractured sternum, fractured scapula or fractured upper ribs
- Differing blood pressures in the arms (as the aorta divides)
- Widened mediastinum on the chest x-ray.

Immediate treatment:

- High flow oxygen
- Establish venous access and send blood for grouping and cross matching
- JUDICIOUS use of intravenous fluids – raising this patient's blood pressure could cause the adventitia to rupture[1]
- Seek senior expert help early, the patient will need a CT scan, blood pressure control to avoid hypertension, angiography and surgery.

Tracheobronchial tree injury

Injury to the trachea and bronchi are suggestive of major blunt force.[7] Most of the injuries occur close to the carina (where the right and left main bronchus meet)[2,4] and are often fatal at the scene of the incident. Air leaking from the injured trachea or bronchi inhibits effective ventilation and the patient becomes hypoxic.

Signs and symptoms suggestive of a tracheobronchial tree injury:

- Respiratory distress, cough or haemoptysis in the conscious patient
- Subcutaneous emphysema (air leaking into the surrounding tissues)
- Pneumothorax that doesn't respond to tube thoracostomy (because of the continued air leak from the injury).

Immediate treatment:

- High flow oxygen
- Call for senior expert help – intubation may be very difficult due to swelling or bleeding in the trachea[1,2,4]
- The patient may need to go for urgent bronchoscopy or surgery to confirm the diagnosis and repair the injury.

Oesophageal perforation

Injury to the oesophagus is usually caused by a penetrating force.[2] The object enters the neck or thorax, causing a hole in the oesophagus from which stomach contents can escape into the thorax.[1]

Signs and symptoms suggestive of oesophageal perforation:

- A penetrating chest or neck wound
- Shocked patient
- Chest pain/epigastric pain
- Haemetemesis
- Subcutaneous emphysema.

Immediate treatment:

- High flow oxygen
- Establish venous access and send blood for grouping and cross matching
- Urgent surgical referral
- Intravenous antibiotics may be needed because the gastric contents leak causing infection.

Myocardial contusion

Case study 4.2 Blunt chest injury

A 69-year-old female is involved in an RTA. She is the driver of a small car that has gone into the back of a stationary lorry at approximately 35 mph. Unfortunately the patient was not wearing a seat belt. On arrival to the ED she has high flow oxygen in situ, two large bore cannulae have been inserted by the paramedics and her vital signs are:

RR 19, HR 121, BP 156/99

She is complaining of neck pain and has cervical spine immobilisation in situ. She is also complaining of chest pain and difficulty in breathing and has a large contusion over her sternum. Clinical examination does not find any sources of haemorrhage however she has decreased air entry on the left. Her chest x-ray shows a fracture to the sternum and single fractures to ribs 4, 6 and 7 on the left side of the chest.

A chest drain is inserted into her left chest with no blood loss. The tube is swinging and a further chest x-ray confirms the tube is in the correct position. However, the patient is becoming progressively tachycardic and the cardiac monitor shows a number of ventricular ectopics. A 12 lead ECG is performed which shows myocardial ischaemia. A diagnosis of myocardial contusion is made and the patient is urgently referred to the on call cardiologists.

Bruising or contusion of the heart is caused by blunt trauma and suggests a severe force was involved, such as direct impact or compression. Myocardial contusion is often associated with fractures of the sternum,[1] thoracic spine or rib fractures.[2]

Signs and symptoms suggestive of a myocardial contusion:

- Injury to the sternum, thoracic spine or ribs
- Chest pain
- Cardiac arrhythmias such as sinus tachycardia, narrow complex tachycardia, ventricular ectopics
- Signs of myocardial ischaemia – ST changes, bundle branch block.

Immediate treatment:

- 12 lead ECG and continuous cardiac monitoring
- Close observation of pulse and blood pressure
- Referral to cardiology – the patient may need an echocardiogram.

Pulmonary contusion

Pulmonary contusion is the most common, potentially lethal thoracic injury.[2,4] Any patient with a significant chest wall or rib injury is at risk of developing pulmonary contusion. The lung tissue is damaged, resulting in bleeding, bruising and pulmonary oedema. This impairs normal ventilation and gaseous exchange and the patient becomes hypoxic.

Signs and symptoms suggestive of pulmonary contusion:

- Blunt injury to the chest wall or rib fractures
- Poor oxygen saturations
- Haemoptysis
- Hypoxia on arterial blood gas results (e.g. PaO_2 of <8 kPa).

Immediate treatment:

- High flow oxygen
- Close monitoring of oxygen saturations and arterial blood gases
- Analgesia to help the patient breathe more comfortably
- JUDICIOUS use of intravenous fluids to avoid exacerbating pulmonary oedema
- Endotracheal intubation and ventilation if the patient is becoming hypoxic.

Diaphragmatic rupture
Diaphragmatic tear or rupture can be caused by blunt or penetrating force to the thorax and/or abdomen. This is discussed in further detail in Chapter 6.

PRIMARY SURVEY ASSESSMENT AND RESUSCITATION

Airway with cervical spine control
As for all trauma patients, assessment of the airway with simultaneous cervical spine control is the first priority for the patient with a thoracic injury. Any patient with an upper thoracic injury must be expected to have a cervical spine injury until proven otherwise by a senior clinician. The neck should be examined for signs of obvious injury such as wounds, swelling or subcutaneous emphysema.

In the conscious patient, hoarseness or coughing may be indicative of an upper thoracic airway injury. This patient should be closely monitored and their airway assessed by a senior anaesthetist.

Systematic assessment and management of the airway is discussed in detail in Chapter 2.

Breathing and ventilation
Application of high flow oxygen 15 L/min via a non-rebreathe mask is the first priority in this stage of the assessment. Following this, the patient's chest should be fully exposed to

allow for systematic assessment of the chest. Using the *look, listen, feel* approach, signs and symptoms of an underlying thoracic injury may be detected:

Look

- Is the patient breathing? Is assisted ventilation with a bag/valve/mask device required?
- Respiratory rate – is the patient tachypnoeic?
- Respiratory depth – are the breaths adequate or more shallow than would be expected?
- Increased work of breathing – use of accessory muscles?
- Symmetry – are both sides of the chest moving equally? (this may be easier viewed from the foot of the patient's bed).
- Paradoxical breathing – is there a deformity or instability in chest movement?
- Look . . . at the oxygen saturation monitor, is the patient hypoxic?
- Wounds – are there signs of wounds, abrasions, bruising or seat belt marks? (anterior and posterior aspects of the chest).
- Is there a significant wound that needs to be covered with a three-sided dressing?

Listen

- Are there obvious sounds heard on inspiration or expiration, e.g. stridor or wheeze?
- On auscultation, can equal breath sounds be heard in all areas?

Feel

- Is the patient complaining of any pain, tenderness in the thoracic region?
- Is there any crepitus, bony tenderness or surgical emphysema detected during gentle examination?

- Percussion may be performed by an experienced clinician to elicit whether there is hypo- or hyperresonance.

Following assessment, if a thoracic injury is suspected:

- Seek senior medical assistance (or the trauma team depending on local protocols)
- Request a chest x-ray – preferably an erect chest x-ray once the cervical spine has been cleared as many injuries are not easily seen on a supine film[8]
- Request arterial blood gas analysis.

CIRCULATION AND HAEMORRHAGE CONTROL

Assessment of the patient's circulatory status is important due to the risk of hypovolaemia and cardiac arrhythmias associated with thoracic injury. The assessment should include:

- Heart rate, regularity and quality – is the patient tachycardic? Is the pulse irregular or suggestive of a cardiac arrhythmia?
- Level of consciousness – is the patient hypoxic, or hypovolaemic and therefore not perfusing their brain properly? Do not dismiss an altered level of consciousness being due to alcohol or drugs.
- Blood pressure – is the patient hypo- or hypertensive? In the presence of a TDA hypertension could cause a rupture of the adventitia.
- Capillary refill time – is the patient peripherally shut down indicating significant shock?
- In the conscious patient, is there any chest pain? Does the patient need an ECG?

Two large bore cannulae should be inserted and blood taken as per trauma protocols (see Chapter 2). All patients over the age of 40 should have an ECG performed and all patients who have sustained a thoracic injury should be connected to a cardiac monitor to detect possible arrhythmias.[3]

If available, a FAST scan should be performed (see Chapter 6 for more detail of this type of scan) to look for the presence of a cardiac tamponade. The patient may need a CT scan to detect more subtle thoracic injuries, however this is preferable in stable patients.

Intravenous fluids for the patient with a thoracic injury

If a significant haemorrhage is suspected in the patient with a thoracic injury, intravenous fluids may be prescribed (see Chapter 2). The following conditions require careful fluid administration as the patient's status can be worsened by aggressive use of intravenous fluids:[1]

- Pulmonary contusion – injury to the lung tissue causes an inflammatory response. Capillaries become leaky, causing fluid to shift into the tissues and alveoli resulting in oedema. Aggressive fluid resuscitation may exacerbate the pulmonary oedema.
- TDA – increasing the blood pressure by fluid resuscitation may cause the adventitia layer to rupture. This will result in uncontrollable haemorrhage and death.

The priority for the cardiovascularly unstable patient is to call for expert help, find the source of the bleeding and control the haemorrhage.

Disability and dysfunction

Assessment of level of the patient's consciousness should be ongoing. Decreased conscious levels may be due to a concurrent head injury or the presence of alcohol or drugs. However, with thoracic injury, an altered level of consciousness must lead to a suspicion of hypoxia and hypovolaemia and the patient investigated for such accordingly.

Exposure and environment control

The patient should be fully undressed to facilitate a through examination and log rolled to ensure that posterior thoracic injuries are not missed. The axillae and the base of the neck should be examined for small penetrating wounds. If not already considered, a urinary catheter should be inserted to monitor urine output.

INDICATIONS FOR A THORACOTOMY IN THE ED

The best place for any major surgical intervention is in an operating theatre. There are a small number of occasions however where emergency thoracic operative procedures take place in the ED or at the scene of the incident. Emergency thoracotomy is performed to clamp great vessels such as the aorta and prevent overwhelming haemorrhage. It is associated with a high mortality and is best performed by an experienced surgeon.[1] Some pre-hospital care doctors have been taught to perform the procedure at scene[9,10] where successful outcomes have been seen when the appropriate patient was chosen (i.e. penetrating injury compared to blunt injury). There is no 'gold standard' recommendation for ED thoracotomy, however the following parameters may be considered:[9]

Penetrating thoracic injury:

- Witnessed cardiac arrest with immediate surgical access
- Unresponsive hypotension (systolic BP <70 mmHg).

Survival following emergency thoracotomy for a stab wound is much higher than for a gunshot wound.[11]

Blunt thoracic injury:

- Unresponsive hypotension (systolic BP <70 mmHg)
- Rapid blood loss form the chest drain (>1500 ml stat).

Emergency thoracotomy for blunt injury is associated with a very low survival rate.[11]

CONCLUSION

Thoracic injuries are common following trauma and can be life threatening. Complex anatomy within the chest means that many structures can be injured resulting in hypoxia, hypovolaemia or a combination of the two. Blunt and penetrating trauma can cause injuries that are immediately life threatening. However, there are a number of injuries that may not be obvious in the initial stages of care in the ED but nevertheless are just as harmful. Systematic assessment, early oxygenation and timely intervention of senior expert help are essential.

KEY INFORMATION BOX

- Beware the patient with a reduced level of consciousness. In thoracic injury this indicates hypoxia and shock!
- Patients who are cardiovascularly unstable need a surgical evaluation urgently
- Penetrating objects must be left in situ until a surgeon has assessed the injury
- Flail chests can cause pulmonary oedema – monitor the oxygen saturations and arterial blood gases
- Patient with multiple rib fractures need adequate analgesia to allow for effective breathing
- A tension pneumothorax does not always cause a deviated trachea – tachycardia and tachypnoea are more urgent signs
- Cover chest wall wounds with a three-sided dressing until an open pneumothorax has been ruled out
- Beware the patient that has a fractured sternum, scapulae or upper ribs fractures – what is their underlying injury?
- Aggressive fluid resuscitation may worsen the outcome for the patient with a thoracic injury.

REFERENCES

1. Greaves I, Porter KM, Ryan JM (Eds) (2001) Head injuries. In: Trauma care manual, 54–70. Arnold, London
2. Pryor JP, Schwab CW, Peitzman AB (2002) Thoracic injury. In: The trauma manual (2nd edn) (Eds Peitzman AB, Rhodes M, Schwab CW, Yealy DM, Fabian TC), 203–235. Lippincott, Williams & Wilkins, Philadelphia
3. Sharpe T, Steyn RS (2005) Cardiothoracic trauma. In: Principles and practice of trauma nursing (Ed O'Shea R), 363–378. Elsevier, Edinburgh

4. American College of Surgeons Committee on Trauma (2004) Thoracic trauma. In: Advanced trauma life support for doctors. Student course manual (7th edn), 103–115. American College of Surgeons, Chicago

5. Leigh-Smith S, Harris T (2005) Tension pneumothorax – time for a re-think? Emergency Medical Journal 22:8–16

6. Ivatury RR (2004) The injured heart. In: Trauma (Eds Moore EE, Feliciano DV, Mattox KL) (5th edn), 555–568. McGraw-Hill, New York

7. American College of Surgeons Committee on Trauma (2004) Biomechanics of injury. In: Advanced trauma life support for doctors. Student course manual (7th edn), 315–335. American College of Surgeons, Chicago

8. Hodgetts T, Turner L (2006) Trauma rules 2 (2nd edn), 108. Blackwell Publishing, Oxford

9. Hodgetts T, Turner L (2006) Trauma rules 2 (2nd edn), 35. Blackwell Publishing, Oxford

10. Wright KD, Murphy K (2002) Cardiac tamponade: a case of kitchen floor thoracotomy. Emergency Medical Journal 19:587–588

11. Brohi K (2006) Emergency department thoracotomy. http://www.trauma.org/index.php/main/article/361

5 | Spinal Injuries

Elaine Cole

INTRODUCTION

Spinal trauma leading to spinal cord injury (SCI) can have devastating life limiting effects. Whilst still a relatively rare injury, the incidence of traumatic SCI in Britain is 10–15 million of the population,[1,2] which equates to approximately 1000 people per year.[3]

The main causes of SCI in Britain are blunt trauma, with falls, followed by road traffic accidents (RTA) being the most common mechanisms of injury. Up to 50% of patients with an SCI also sustain multiple injuries.[3] Penetrating injury to the neck is rare but its incidence appears to be on the increase in urban settings. Whilst any age of patient is susceptible to a SCI during multi-trauma, acute SCI primarily affects young males with an age range of 18–35 years.[4] However, complications of SCI occur with greater frequency in children and older people than any other age group.[3]

SCI can be difficult to detect in the early stages. Any patient who has suffered from a traumatic injury must be suspected of having a SCI until proven otherwise. This is especially important for the patient with a head injury, who is unconscious, has multiple injuries or under the influence of alcohol or drugs where assessment may be more difficult.

The aim of this chapter is to understand the principles of rapid assessment, resuscitation and stabilisation of the person with a spinal cord injury.

LEARNING OBJECTIVES

By the end of this chapter the reader will be able to:

❏ Identify the anatomy of the spine and the spinal cord

❏ Describe the mechanism of spinal injuries
❏ Understand primary and secondary spinal cord injury
❏ Differentiate between spinal shock and neurogenic shock
❏ Describe assessment and management priorities in relation to ABCDE.

ANATOMY OF THE SPINE AND CORD

The spinal column
The spinal column comprises (Figure 5.1):

- 7 cervical vertebrae (C1–C7)
- 12 thoracic vertebrae (T1–T12)
- 5 lumbar vertebrae (L1–L5)
- 5 fused sacral vertebrae (S1–S5).

In between the cervical, thoracic and lumbar vertebrae are intervertebral discs and facet joints. Stabilising ligaments at the front (anterior) and the back (posterior) of the spinal column help to maintain spinal alignment and stability.

For many reasons the cervical spine is most vulnerable to injury.[5] It is a straight, flexible part of the spine, especially in the upper area beneath the occiput (the head). Beneath the level of the third cervical vertebrae (C3) the diameter of the spinal canal (the hole in the vertebrae where the spinal cord runs) is small. Here, the proximity of the spinal cord means that dislocation or fracture of the bony vertebrae can impinge on the cord causing a SCI.

The spinal cord
The spinal cord is a continuation of the brainstem (the medulla).[6] It travels through the vertebral canal, finishing approximately at L1 (the first lumbar vertebrae). The spinal cord is divided into 31 segments, each segment with a pair of nerve roots.[1] Each nerve root innervates (or stimulates):

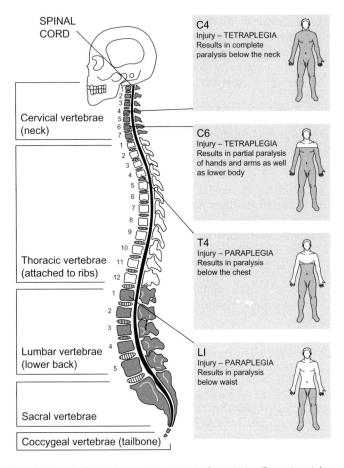

Fig. 5.1 Level of spinal injury and extent of paralysis. (Reproduced from Harrison *et al.* Managing Spinal Cord Injury: the first 48 hours, 2nd edition (2007) with permission from Claire MacDonald/SIA)

- Sensory (feeling) nerves in specific areas of the skin (dermatomes), and
- Motor (movement) nerves in specific muscles (myotomes).

When a spinal cord injury is suspected, an experienced clinician should test sensory and motor function. This is done by examining movement, touch/feeling and reflexes, and abnormalities found during the examination may indicate the level of nerve (neurological) damage.

MECHANISM OF SPINAL CORD INJURY

Blunt trauma
Excessive movement of the spine can be caused by:

- Falls
- Road traffic accidents
- Sporting injuries – rugby, horse riding
- Diving – especially into shallow water
- Self harm (hanging)
- Assault.

Forces that are produced from the excessive movement can cause injury to the spinal cord. Fractures of the vertebral column or injury to the ligaments that stabilise the spine can cause a SCI. If the injury is unstable, causing the bony structure of the spinal column to move, this can result in damage to the spinal cord. Table 5.1 summarises the specific movements sustained during a traumatic event that can injure the spinal column and potentially the spinal cord.[1,4,6]

Penetrating trauma
Penetrating trauma to the neck, such as stabbing, shooting or impalement, can cause a number of injuries.[7,8] The location of airway, vascular, nerve and digestive tract structures within the neck mean that any penetrating wound needs to be carefully examined by an experienced clinician.

The neck is divided into three anatomical zones (Figure 5.2), which indicate the structures that may be involved:[7,8]

- Zone 1 is from the clavicles to the cricoid cartilage. The trachea, oesophagus, upper mediastinum and upper portion of the lungs are within this zone.

Table 5.1 Spinal column movements caused by blunt force

Movement	Resulting injury
Hyperflexion	The spine bending sharply forward can cause destabilisation of the posterior ligaments. This allows movement of the vertebrae, which may damage the spinal cord
Hyperflexion with rotation	50–80% of cervical spine injuries and most thoracolumbar injuries are caused by these movements. The spine bending sharply forward and at the same time rotating can severely disrupt the posterior ligaments and may fracture or dislocate the vertebrae
Hyperextension	This is where the head is forced backwards (e.g. when striking the head on a steering wheel or step) causing disruption to the anterior stabilising ligaments. The posterior aspect of the bony structures may be fractured. A C2/C3 injury caused this way is common in hanging
Compression	Compression can be due to direct force crushing the spinal column or by hyperflexion causing the vertebral body to be compressed and fracture. Thoracolumbar fractures are common with this mechanism
Axial loading	This is a type of compression. Axial loading is caused by a heavy weight falling onto the head, landing on the head after a fall or hitting the head on the roof of a car when unrestrained. Fractures of C1 (the atlas) – known as Jefferson's fractures and C2 (the axis) are common with this mechanism

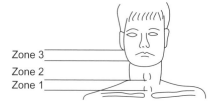

Fig. 5.2 Zones of penetrating neck injury

- Zone 2 is from the cricoid cartilage to the angle of the mandible. The carotid and vertebral arteries, jugular veins, oesophagus, trachea, pharynx and larynx are within this zone.
- Zone 3 is from the angle of the mandible to the base of the skull. The carotid and vertebral arteries and jugular veins are within this zone.

Whilst penetrating neck injuries may cause airway and bleeding problems, there is a risk that the penetrating object can injure the vertebrae in the cervical spine or pass through the vertebral canal damaging the cord. This may result in a complete or incomplete SCI. Therefore, patients with a penetrating neck injury should be immobilised and assessed as for any spinal trauma patient.

PRIMARY AND SECONDARY SCI

SCI can be divided into primary and secondary injuries. Primary injury refers to the injury that has occurred at the time of the incident. Secondary injury occurs minutes or hours after the primary injury and it is the health care professional's role to minimise the risk of this.

Primary SCI

As described in the mechanism of injury section above, a number of excessive movements or penetrating object can injure the spine. The force that occurs can cause:

- Fractures
- Dislocation
- Subluxation (partial dislocation)
- Haematoma formation
- Soft tissue swelling.

All of these injuries can damage spinal cord, by reducing blood supply to the cord or affecting the structure of the cord. Primary SCI can vary in severity. A complete transection of the spinal cord will result in death. Partial injury to the spinal cord may be temporary or permanent depending on the amount of swelling and cord tissue ischaemia that develops.[4]

Secondary SCI

Secondary injury occurs as the injured spinal cord continues to swell, or surrounding structures such as bone or haematoma continue to compress the cord. This secondary injury can be worsened by the following:[2,4]

- Mechanical instability
- Hypoxia
- Hypoperfusion.

Mechanical instability

The patient with an SCI should be carefully handled and positioned to avoid further damage.[1] In-line immobilisation should be maintained to minimise the risk of destabilising the spinal injury. When being moved for examination of the back, placement of sliding sheets or relief of pressure areas, the patient should be log rolled using four people (see Chapter 2).

Hypoxia

Hypoxia in trauma can be caused by lung injury, haemorrhage or poor respiratory effort due to a head injury. *However, a SCI can also cause hypoxia.*

Injuries to the cervical spine at C3–C4 can cause damage to the phrenic nerve causing paralysis of the diaphragm. If the diaphragm is affected the patient's breathing may become laboured, with paradoxical movement (where the chest and abdomen appear to move at different times), and be more shallow than normal. These patients will usually require mechanical ventilation.[4]

Other respiratory problems can occur for patients with cervical and upper thoracic spinal injuries. In these parts of the spine the intercostal muscles are innervated.[9] If the nerves that supply these muscles are damaged then the ability to breathe deeply and cough will be affected. Careful observation of the patient's respiratory effort is needed and ventilatory support may be required.

Hypoperfusion

The major cause of secondary SCI is disruption of the blood flow to the spinal cord.[6] This can be caused by direct vessel injury in the spinal column or because the patient is hypovolaemic due to another bleeding problem (e.g. pelvic fracture, liver injury). If the spinal cord is allowed to become *hypoperfused* its function will be reduced and eventually cell death of the spinal cord tissue will occur, leading to more permanent disability.

Minimising movement of the patient and treatment of hypovolaemia will help to prevent hypoperfusion of the cord.[4]

SPINAL SHOCK AND NEUROGENIC SHOCK

In SCI the terms 'spinal shock' and 'neurogenic shock' are sometimes used interchangeably. They are however not the same, and should not be confused with each other.[10]

Spinal shock

Spinal shock can be defined as a complete loss of all neurological function, including reflexes and rectal tone, below the level of the SCI.[2,4] It is a transient condition, caused by swelling of the cord following an injury. Spinal shock has been described as being similar to 'concussion' of the spinal cord.[1] Below the level of the SCI there will be loss of sensation (feeling) and movement, resulting in a flaccid paralysis. In male patients there is sometimes an involuntary priapism.[10]

Spinal shock can last hours to several weeks,[1] and only after the swelling around the spinal cord has subsided can the SCI be assessed to decide if it is temporary or permanent.

Neurogenic shock

Neurogenic shock is caused by damage to the sympathetic pathways in the spinal cord.[5] The sympathetic nervous system pathways exit the thoracic spine at the level of T6. Neurogenic shock, therefore, usually does not occur in injuries below T6.[2]

Damage to the sympathetic pathways can cause alteration to normal autonomic function:

- Loss of vasomotor tone
- Loss of sympathetic innervation to the heart.

Loss of vasomotor tone

The sympathetic nervous system helps to control the muscle tone in the blood vessels (known as vasomotor tone) in the lower extremities and abdominal viscera. If the vasomotor tone is lost because of sympathetic pathway damage, the blood vessels will not be able to constrict, instead vasodilation will occur. This will cause pooling of the blood in the vessels and consequently hypotension.[5]

Loss of sympathetic innervation to the heart

Case study 5.1 Neurogenic shock

A 32-year-old male is being assessed in the ED. He was involved in an RTA, an unrestrained back seat passenger, when the car he was travelling in collided with a lorry. He has sustained head and face injuries and has been intubated to protect his airway. The nurse involved in his care notes that his pulse is stable but he is becoming hypotensive:

RR 14 (ventilated), HR 77, BP 94/60

The patient has a chest x-ray, which indicates a right-sided haemothorax and the FAST scan shows bleeding around the liver. A chest drain is inserted and he is prepared for theatre. He is becoming progressively hypotensive, however his pulse remains normal. The nursing and medical students watching the trauma call ask why the patient has not become tachycardic if he is bleeding internally. They are told that he has developed neurogenic shock.

Table 5.2 Comparison of hypovolaemic shock with neurogenic shock

Parameter	Hypovolaemic shock	Neurogenic shock
Pulse rate	Raised	Normal
Blood pressure	Normal at first, lowered in later stages of shock	Lowered
Skin	Pale, cool, clammy	Normal, warm, flushed

The sympathetic nervous system helps to innervate the heart, causing tachycardia as a response to haemorrhage, fear or pain. In neurogenic shock, the sympathetic pathways have been damaged, therefore if the patient is bleeding, there will not be a tachycardia as would normally be expected.

Hypovolaemic shock is much more common that neurogenic shock.[9] If a patient is hypotensive, it is much safer to suspect hypovolaemic shock and try to detect a source of bleeding rather than presume the low blood pressure is due to a spinal injury.

Table 5.2 illustrates some of the differences between hypovolaemic and neurogenic shock.

PRIMARY SURVEY ASSESSMENT AND RESUSCITATION

The patient with a potential SCI should be assessed systematically as for any trauma patient. Many patients with a SCI also have major injuries,[2] therefore evaluation of the spine can be deferred until assessment for life-threatening injuries has been completed.[1] By resuscitating the whole patient the spine will benefit.

Airway and cervical spine

The airway must be assessed whilst keeping the spine in alignment. If the patient has an obstructed airway then a jaw thrust manoeuvre should be used without flexing the neck. An unconscious patient should have their airway secured with endotracheal intubation, as described in Chapter 2.

Case study 5.2 Vagal nerve stimulation during intubation

A 21-year-old male has sustained a cervical spinal cord injury from diving into shallow water. He is becoming progressively less responsive and his respiratory effort is decreasing. The senior doctor in charge of his care decides that the patient should be intubated and ventilated to protect his airway and support his breathing.

The ED nurse and operating department practitioner (ODP) assist the anaesthetist to intubate the patient. The ODP applies cricoid pressure whilst the nurse administers the anaesthetic drugs. As the anaesthetist inserts the endotracheal tube the nurse notes that the patient's heart rate has slowed to 41 from 80. This is reported to the anaesthetist who requests that the patient be given intravenous atropine immediately.

During airway management, use of suction or insertion of the endotracheal tube can cause vagus nerve stimulation. When the vagus nerve, (part of which is situated in the neck) gets stimulated there is a slowing of the heart rate (bradycardia). In a non-spinal injured patient this would not be a problem, as the sympathetic response would return the heart rate to normal. However, in a patient with a cervical or high thoracic injury where there is damage to the spinal pathways (see above) there will not be an automatic correction of the brady-cardia. Therefore when suctioning or intubating the patient with a SCI, atropine 0.5–1 mg (a drug that blocks the vagus nerve) should be available in case the patient becomes bradycardic.

Cervical spine immobilisation
Cervical spine immobilisation should continue throughout the patient assessment. Immobilisation should consist of:

- Application of a correctly sized semi-rigid collar, and manual immobilisation, or
- Application of a correctly sized semi-rigid collar, head blocks and straps.

If the patient has wounds or external injuries to the neck, a collar can still be applied. Sterile gauze or a non-adherent dressing can be used to loosely cover the wound beneath the collar. A heavily bleeding wound may need to have direct pressure applied and the wound explored by a senior doctor urgently.

Patients should not be left on a rigid spinal board or ambulance scoop stretcher once they arrive in the ED. Many patients are left on spinal boards unnecessarily.[6] These devices are very uncomfortable and can cause increased pressure to the buttocks, sacrum, back and shoulders. If left on one of these devices the patient may become restless and agitated, and this may result in movement, which could aggravate any existing spinal injury. Other causes of restlessness and agitation include:

- Hypoxia
- Hypovolaemia
- A concurrent head injury
- Alcohol or drugs
- Medication (such as ketamine or morphine)
- Pain
- Nausea/the need to vomit
- Fear.

An agitated, confused patient *should not be immobilised* if this increases the agitation and causes potentially harmful movement. The goal here is to:

- Find out *why the patient is agitated*
- Treat the cause
- Apply immobilisation when the patient is calmer.

In emergency situations, the use of a sedative or paralysing agent may be used, however this requires considerable clinical judgement, skill and expertise.[2]

A conscious patient with severe facial injuries with a lot of associated bleeding may not want to lie flat. The injury and bleeding may cause an airway obstruction if the patient is forced to lie down.[7] Whilst the patient is conscious it is preferable to allow them to sit upright with a semi-rigid collar in situ and request senior medical help to assess the patient urgently.

The immobilised patient who is nauseated or vomiting

It can be very distressing for the immobilised patient who feels nauseated. It is not 'normal' to vomit whilst lying flat and the patient may feel frightened or start to panic about choking. An antiemetic should be administered as a matter of urgency. If the immobilised patient needs to vomit, do one of two things:

Rapidly gather four people to carry out a log roll. The patient can then vomit whilst on their side. A fifth person should be available to assist and support the patient.

OR

If four people are not available, tilt the bed or trolley head down. If the patient vomits, the vomitus will flow away from the face and head. This is very unpleasant for the patient however it minimises the risk of choking and aspiration. Remove the rigid suction catheter from the suction tubing and use the wide bore suction tubing to clear the secretions.

Breathing and ventilation

To avoid hypoxia and thus minimise the risk of secondary SCI, high flow oxygen 15 L/min should be administered early. Box 5.1 re-iterates the causes of hypoxia in a SCI. Additionally underlying lung injury such as a haemothorax or pulmonary contusion can cause hypoxia. In order to detect breathing problems due to a SCI, assessment of breathing and ventilation should include:

- Respiratory rate
- Respiratory effort – depth and use of accessory muscles

> **Box 5.1 Respiratory compromise caused by a spinal injury**
>
> • Patients with a cervical spine injury are at risk of phrenic nerve impairment, which may result in diaphragmatic paralysis
> • Patients with higher thoracic spine injury are at risk of intercostal nerve paralysis

• Oxygen saturations
• Arterial blood gas measurement in the unwell patient.

A patient who is tiring, unable to take 'normal' deep breaths or is unable to cough fully may be developing breathing problems related to a SCI. This should be reported to a senior clinician urgently as the patient may need to be intubated and ventilated.

Circulation and haemorrhage control

Assessment of circulation should be carried out as for any trauma patient. *Remember that SCI can mask the signs and symptoms of internal haemorrhage.*

Vital signs should be recorded frequently, including:

• Heart rate
• Blood pressure
• Capillary refill time
• Level of consciousness.

Damage to the sympathetic pathways in the spinal cord may mean that the normal characteristics of hypovolaemic shock, such as tachycardia and pale, vasoconstricted skin, are not present. Absence of such signs does not mean that the patient is not bleeding somewhere!

Hypotension should be regarded as a sign of:

• Thoracic bleeding
• Abdominal bleeding

- Pelvic injury
- External haemorrhage.

before considering neurogenic shock.[3] If the patient is hypotensive, a search for the possible sources of bleeding must be made, using clinical examination and a FAST scan. Remember that the shock may be both hypovolaemic and neurogenic.[6]

If a source of bleeding is found then the patient should be referred to the appropriate surgical team for definitive care. If no source of bleeding is found then the neurogenic shock needs to be treated.

Management of hypotension in neurogenic shock

To avoid hypoperfusion and thus minimise the risk of a secondary SCI, intravenous fluids (crystalloids) need to be given, but with caution. There is a risk that excessive fluid administration may cause pulmonary oedema.[1,2,6] Fluid boli of 250–500 ml may be given, reassessing after each bolus.

A urinary catheter should be inserted to monitor urine output and allow for assessment of the patient's fluid balance. Ultrasonic cardiac output monitoring (if available) may be used to determine the patient's haemodynamic status.[11] Alternatively, central venous pressure monitoring can help to measure the patient's need for fluids.

If the patient's blood pressure fails to respond to intravenous fluids, vasopressors such as noradrenaline may be indicated to raise the blood pressure.[1,2] A senior clinician and local guidelines should be consulted prior to considering this.

Disability and dysfunction

When assessing the conscious patient, the presence of any of the following may indicate a possible SCI:

- Back or neck pain (most conscious patients with a spinal injury will complain of pain)[1]
- Limb weakness
- Altered sensation, such as numbness, pins and needles, tingling.

If the mechanism of injury suggests a SCI and any of the above are present, a senior clinician should carry out a full neurological examination.

The presence of limb weakness, paralysis or loss of sensation may be very distressing for the patient. Spinal injury is an emotive, challenging issue to be dealt with in the ED, especially for staff who have limited experience or knowledge in this area.[4] An honest, sensitive approach is recommended. It is difficult to make predictions about the future with limited information in the early stages of care therefore specialist advice should be sought.

Steroids for patients with a SCI

Management of acute SCI has included the use of steroids, namely methylprednisolone, for the past 30 years, with many studies examining its efficacy.[6] The drug acts by reducing the inflammation and oedema that occurs following an injury to the spinal cord. Its use, however, is not without risk. Following the use of methylprednisolone in multiply injured patients there have been reports of:[6]

- Sepsis
- Pulmonary oedema
- Gastrointestinal disturbances following the use of methylprednisolone.

Despite many studies demonstrating benefits and risks, evidence of potential harm from steroids in SCI far outweighs the evidence of potential improvement and the use can no longer be justified.[12]

Exposure and environmental control

The patient's clothes should be removed and the patient should be carefully log rolled to allow for examination of the back. A senior clinician may examine the rectal sphincter for tone as part of the neurological assessment.

An undressed patient is at risk of developing hypothermia. This may be worsened if the patient is in neurogenic shock and has loss of vasomotor tone. Vasodilation may occur causing heat loss through the skin, therefore once the examination is completed, the patient should be covered.

Some patients with a SCI lose the ability to control their own temperature. This is known as poikilothermia, and the patient assumes the temperature of the surrounding environment.[4] This should be taken into account in very warm or cool clinical environments or when transferring the patient for example.

Clearing the cervical spine

Patients who do not have any spinal pain or neurological deficit may not require x-rays. A decision making tool, such as the Canadian C-Spine Rules, can be used to help make that decision.[13] This comprises three main questions and suggests that a patient may not require x-rays if:

- There is no high risk factor present that mandates radiography (i.e. age ≥65 years, dangerous mechanism or paraesthesia in extremities)
- There are any low risk factors present that allow safe assessment of range of motion (i.e. simple rear-end motor vehicle collision, sitting position in ED, ambulatory at any time since injury, delayed onset of neck pain, or absence of midline C-spine tenderness)
- The patient is able to actively rotate neck 45° to the left and right.

The cervical spine may be clinically cleared and the collar removed if the patient fulfils certain criteria. For example, the NEXUS guidelines[7] suggest that the cervical spine can be cleared clinically if:

- The patient has a GCS of 15 *and*
- There is no posterior midline cervical tenderness *and*
- There is no focal neurological deficit *and*
- There is no intoxication from alcohol, drugs and prescribed medications.

Local policy should be followed before implementing these guidelines.

DIAGNOSTIC IMAGING FOR THE SPINAL INJURED PATIENT

If a spinal injury is suspected due to pain, altered neurological function or mechanism of injury, the role of good quality imaging is crucial.

In the ED initially this usually means x-rays. For the cervical spine a lateral film and an AP (anterior posterior) film should be taken. It is essential that the whole of the cervical spine is included from C1 through to T1, to ensure that upper and lower injuries are not missed.[3,4,7]

CT scanning can be used to examine the bones with accurate detail.[4] In the unconscious patient following blunt trauma, CT scanning has been shown to detect cervical spine injuries much more accurately than plain x-rays.[14] MRI scanning, if available, can identify cord damage, haematomas, ligamentous injury and oedema surrounding the injury.[1,3,4]

SCIWORA

There are a small number of patients, usually unconscious following blunt trauma, who have a neurological deficit without bony injury being detected on an x-ray. This is known as SCIWORA: Spinal Cord Injury WithOut Radiological Abnormality.[7] The patient should be kept immobilised and specialist advice sought from a neurosurgeon.

DEFINITIVE CARE FOR THE SPINAL INJURED PATIENT

The ongoing care that the patient with a spinal injury will receive depends on the injury sustained, treatment needed and resources available. Some patients may need surgery, which should be carried out by a neurosurgeon or orthopaedic surgeon with an interest in spinal injuries. Patients may need to go to the intensive care setting for ventilation and specialist therapies input.

Specialist advice should be sought early to ensure the best patient care. The Spinal Injuries Association suggests that all NHS hospitals should have a common protocol for the care of the patient with a SCI using knowledge and expertise from a spinal injury unit (SIU).[4] This protocol, drawn up between the hospital and the SIU, should detail the specialist care that the patient may need before transfer to the SIU.

CONCLUSION

Spinal trauma resulting in spinal cord injuries can provide challenges for ED staff in the early phase of the patient's care. Injury can be caused by blunt or penetrating force. However, signs and symptoms are not always obvious immediately. Mechanical instability, hypoxia and hypoperfusion can worsen the spinal injury. The presence of spinal shock or neurogenic shock can complicate the overall picture of the patient, making it difficult to detect other problems.

Priorities for the patient's care include careful airway management, cervical spine immobilisation, ongoing assessment of breathing and circulation. The psychological impact of a spinal injury can be immense for the conscious patient. Honest, sensitive care is required. Early specialist input is essential to ensure that the patient has optimal care and treatment.

KEY INFORMATION BOX

- Any patient who has sustained multiple injuries must be suspected of having a spinal injury until proven otherwise
- An agitated or confused patient should not be forced into cervical spine immobilisation – FIND THE CAUSE OF THE AGITATION
- Spinal injury can be worsened by mechanical instability, hypoxia and hypoperfusion
- Be suspicious of the patient who is tiring, has shallow breaths or has difficulty coughing
- Spinal shock is where the cord is swollen and 'concussed' and the patient loses feeling and movement below the level of the injury

- Neurogenic shock is where there is impairment to the sympathetic pathways
- Hypotension should suggest hypovolaemic shock rather than neurogenic shock – GET EXPERT HELP TO FIND THE HAEMORRHAGE
- Access specialist help if a SCI is suspected or detected.

REFERENCES

1. Gallagher SM (2005) Spinal trauma. In: Principles and practice of trauma nursing (Ed O'Shea R), 421–429. Elsevier, Edinburgh
2. Fraser MH (2005) Management of acute spinal injury. In: Critical care focus 11: Trauma (Ed Galley H), 36–51. Blackwell Publishing, Oxford
3. Harrison P, Inman C, Williams S (2007) Causes on SCI. In: Managing spinal cord injury: the first 48 hours (2nd edn) (Ed Harrison P), 6–11. Spinal Injuries Association, Milton Keynes
4. Greaves I, Porter KM, Ryan JM (Eds) (2001) Spinal injuries. In: Trauma care manual, 124–141. Arnold, London
5. American College of Surgeons Committee on Trauma (2004) Spine and spinal cord trauma. In: Advanced trauma life support for doctors. Student course manual (7th edn), 177–189. American College of Surgeons, Chicago
6. Welch WC, Donaldson WF, Marion DW (2002) Injuries to the spinal cord and the spinal column. In: The trauma manual (2nd edn) (Eds Peitzman AB, Rhodes M, Schwab CW, Yealy DM, Fabian TC), 140–156. Lippincott, Williams & Wilkins, Philadelphia
7. Maxwell RA (2002) Penetrating neck injury. In: The trauma manual (2nd edn) (Eds Peitzman AB, Rhodes M, Schwab CW, Yealy DM, Fabian TC), 189–197. Lippincott, Williams & Wilkins, Philadelphia
8. Platz A, Kossmann T, Payne B, Trentz O (2003) Stab wounds to the neck with partial transection to the spinal

cord and penetrating injury to the esophagus. Journal of Trauma: Injury, Infection and Critical Care 54:612–614

9. Harrison P, MacKay K, Fletcher A (2007) Systemic effects of spinal cord injury key points: respiratory system. In: Managing spinal cord injury: the first 48 hours (2nd edn) (Ed Harrison P), 67–68. Spinal Injuries Association, Milton Keynes

10. Hodgetts T, Turner L (2006) Trauma rules 2 (2nd edn), 69. Blackwell Publishing, Oxford

11. USCOM (2003) Case studies. http://www.uscom.com.au:80/case_studies.htm

12. Short D, Harrison P (2007) Systemic effects of spinal cord injury key points: neurological system. In: Managing spinal cord injury: the first 48 hours (2nd edn) (Ed Harrison P), 64–66. Spinal Injuries Association, Milton Keynes

13. Steill IG, Wells GA, Vandemheen KL, Clement CM, Lesiuk H, De Maio VJ, Laupacis A, Schull M, McKnight RD, Verbeek R, Brison R, Cass D, Dreyer J, Eisenhauer MA, Greenberg GH, MacPhail I, Morrison L, Reardon M, Worthington J (2001) The Canadian c-spine rule for radiography in alert and stable patients. JAMA 286: 1841–1848

14. Brohi K, Healy M, Fotheringham T, Chan O, Aylwin C, Whitley S, Walsh M (2005) Helical computed tomographic scanning for the evaluation of the cervical spine in the unconscious intubated trauma patient. Journal of Trauma 58:897–901

Abdominal Injuries

Elaine Cole

6

INTRODUCTION

Abdominal injuries account for 20% of trauma related fatalities in the UK each year.[1] Due to the location of the abdomen in the body, injuries resulting from blunt force are rarely isolated and abdominal trauma often involves concurrent chest, pelvic or spinal injuries.[2] Blunt force, such as compression and rapid deceleration, can cause solid abdominal organs to bleed and hollow viscera such as the bowel, to rupture. Penetrating force such as impalement or stab wounds can cause localised abdominal injury, whereas bullets and high velocity missiles can cause more widespread damage throughout the abdominal cavity.

Mortality and morbidity associated with abdominal trauma tends to occur in two stages. In the early stages, rapid uncontrollable or unrecognised haemorrhage can cause hypovolaemic cardiac arrest. Days after the incident, death may occur due to sepsis, disseminated intravascular coagulation, multiorgan failure and abdominal compartment syndrome.[2] The goal for treating patients with abdominal trauma is early recognition of problems and early surgical intervention if necessary, to increase the patient's chances of survival.

The aim of this chapter is to understand the principles of rapid assessment, resuscitation and stabilisation of the person with an abdominal injury.

LEARNING OBJECTIVES

By the end of this chapter the reader will be able to:

❑ Identify abdominal anatomy

❏ Define how blunt and penetrating forces cause differing injury patterns
❏ Identify some specific abdominal injuries
❏ Describe assessment and management priorities in relation to ABCDE
❏ Understand the diagnostic imaging needed to diagnose abdominal injuries.

ABDOMINAL ANATOMY

The abdominal region extends from the 4th intercostal space on full expiration through to the groin and buttock creases. The abdominal region contains many structures that can be affected during traumatic injury:

- The diaphragm, a large muscular structure, separates the thoracic cavity from the abdominal cavity.
- The outer layer of the peritoneum, the parietal peritoneum, lines the wall of the abdominal cavity.
- The inner layer of the peritoneum, the visceral peritoneum, covers some of the intra-abdominal organs.
- The potential space between the layers of the peritoneum is known as the peritoneal cavity. Traumatic injury to the abdomen can cause bleeding to occur within the peritoneal cavity.

The organs situated inside the peritoneum are known as *viscera*. When considering the location of abdominal organs, the abdominal cavity can be divided into four, known as quadrants (Figure 6.1).

Structures located within the Right Upper Quadrant (RUQ):

- Right lobe of the liver
- Gallbladder
- Head of pancreas
- Duodenum
- Sections of the ascending and transverse colon.

Structures located within the Left Upper Quadrant (LUQ):

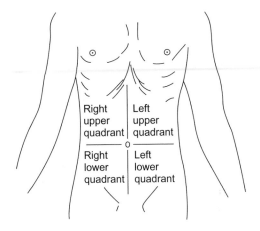

Fig. 6.1 The four quadrants of the abdomen

- Left lobe of the liver
- Stomach
- Spleen
- Body of the pancreas
- Sections of the descending and transverse colon.

Structures located within the Left Lower Quadrant (LLQ):

- Caecum
- Appendix
- Section of the ascending colon.

Structures located within the Right Lower Quadrant (RLQ):

- Sigmoid colon
- Section of the descending colon.

The retroperitonium is the region that is located behind or *posterior* to the peritoneal cavity. Organs such as the kidneys and pancreas, and major vessels including the aorta and the inferior vena cava, are situated within the retroperitonium.

The bladder, prostate gland (in males), rectum and reproductive organs are situated in the pelvic cavity within the bony pelvic ring, and are discussed in more detail in Chapter 7.

MECHANISMS OF ABDOMINAL TRAUMA

Blunt abdominal trauma

The abdomen has little bony protection therefore its contents are susceptible to blunt force.[3] Injury to any of the intra-abdominal structures may occur though blunt force, such as:

- Compression of an organ or viscera against the spine, the pelvis or the abdominal wall
- Direct trauma causing increased pressure and therefore injury to an organ or hollow viscera
- Rapid deceleration causing shearing or tearing of an organ or viscera
- Fractures of lower ribs causing injury to the organ or viscera beneath them.

Penetrating abdominal trauma

Injury may be localised, i.e. in one place, or diffuse (or widespread) depending on the penetrating force. This can be divided into:

- High velocity penetration – rifles, bomb blasts and/or missiles causing cavitation, compression of solid organs and massive wounding
- Low velocity penetration – knives, blades and/or hand guns causing localised injury dependent on the range and the anatomical region affected.

SPECIFIC ABDOMINAL INJURIES

The liver

The liver is situated predominantly in the right upper quadrant and is the most commonly injured solid abdominal organ.[4] It is divided into two lobes, left and right, and is covered completely by a dense connective tissue layer or capsule. The liver lies under the diaphragm and the right lobe is partially located beneath the right lower ribs, therefore damage to the liver should always be suspected with any right lower rib injury. It is a vascular organ, susceptible to haemorrhage as it is supplied with blood by the hepatic arteries and the hepatic portal veins.

Clinical signs and symptoms of liver injury
Any of the following may indicate a liver injury:

- Abrasions, bruising and/or wounds in the right upper quadrant
- Pain in the right upper quadrant or upper abdomen
- Right lower rib fractures
- Signs of hypovolaemic shock/haemodynamic instability.

Diagnosis is made by clinical examination of the abdomen by a senior clinician and diagnostic imaging (discussed later in this chapter). This, together with the cardiovascular status of the patient, will determine whether the treatment of the injury is surgery or conservative management. *In order to detect patient deterioration, it is essential to closely monitor the vital signs such as pulse and blood pressure in the patient with a suspected liver injury.*

The spleen
The spleen is an oval organ that is situated in the left upper quadrant between the fundus (or top) of the stomach and the diaphragm. It is covered in a capsule of dense connective tissue. The spleen is partially located beneath the left lower ribs, therefore damage to the spleen should always be suspected with any left lower rib injury.[4] The spleen is a vascular organ with blood supplied by the splenic arteries, splenic veins and hilar veins (lymphatic vessels) making it susceptible to haemorrhage following injury.

A large proportion of this organ is lymphatic tissue and the functions of the spleen are to develop antibody producing cells and to phagocytose (ingest) bacteria and old red blood cells and platelets. This role in helping the autoimmune system means that patients with splenic injuries who are haemodynamically stable may be treated conservatively wherever possible.

Clinical signs and symptoms of a splenic injury
Any of the following may indicate a splenic injury:

- Abrasions, bruising and/or wounds in the left upper quadrant
- Pain in the left upper quadrant or radiating up to the left shoulder
- Left lower rib fractures
- Signs of hypovolaemic shock/haemodynamic instability.

Diagnosis is made by clinical examination of the abdomen by a senior clinician and diagnostic imaging (discussed later in this chapter). This, together with the cardiovascular status of the patient will determine whether the treatment of the injury is surgery or conservative management. *In order to detect patient deterioration, it is essential to closely monitor the vital signs such as pulse and blood pressure in the patient with a suspected splenic injury.*

The diaphragm
The diaphragm is a large dome shaped muscle divided into two halves (each a *hemi diaphragm*). Its main function is to help with respiration and it is stimulated by the phrenic nerve. Blunt force, such as compression or rapid deceleration, can cause a tear or rupture in the diaphragm. A penetrating force, such as a knife, can cause a wound in the diaphragm. Many penetrating injuries to the left lower thoracic or left upper abdominal regions will involve the left diaphragm.[5]

Clinical signs and symptoms of a diaphragmatic injury
With either mechanism, the size of the injury to the diaphragm will determine the severity of the signs and symptoms experienced by the patient. A small wound or tear may cause some abdominal pain or may be asymptomatic initially. A larger

rupture or perforation may result in the abdominal contents herniating up (pushing upwards) into the chest cavity causing cardiopulmonary compromise as the abdominal organs and viscera compress the thoracic organs.

A number of other clinical signs and symptoms may be present, including:

- Signs of hypovolaemic shock/haemodynamic instability
- Severe abdominal pain
- Abdominal muscle rigidity or *guarding*
- Difficulty in breathing due to lung compromise
- Bowel sounds when auscultating the lungs.

Diagnosis may be made by clinical examination of the abdomen and chest, a FAST scan of the abdomen and a chest x-ray which may show that abdominal contents have been pushed up into the chest cavity. If a nasogastric tube has been passed, on x-ray this may appear to be located in the chest rather than the abdomen. Patients with a diaphragmatic injury need an urgent surgical referral as severe injuries will need careful examination and probable surgery.

The kidneys

The kidneys are situated in the retroperitonium, at the back of the torso, towards the side or flank. Renal injury may be caused by blunt forces such as direct impact or compression, or penetrating forces such as a knife or bullet. Acute life-threatening renal injuries are rare; however, unrecognised renal injury can cause renal failure, which may be life threatening or life limiting.

Any patient who has sustained trauma to the abdomen or back should have urinalysis performed as a routine to look for microscopic haematuria, which may indicate kidney or ureter injury.[4]

Clinical signs and symptoms of a renal injury
The following signs and symptoms may indicate the presence of renal injury:

- Abrasion, contusion and/or wound in the loin region
- Loin pain
- Flank tenderness
- Haematuria.

Diagnosis is made by CT scan using an intravenous dye or *contrast* to show both kidney and ureter structure and function.[1] Most kidney injuries are managed conservatively but a severe injury may result in uncontrolled bleeding that may need an investigative laparotomy and possibly a nephrectomy.

Evisceration

Evisceration occurs when a penetrating force causes a wound in the abdominal wall leading to bowel and omentum (a fold of the peritoneum) protruding or *eviscerating* through the wound.[1] Evisceration can look alarming, however it must not detract from the assessment and resuscitation priorities. *The abdominal contents should not be pushed back into the abdominal cavity as there is a risk of causing further bleeding*. The eviscerated bowel should be covered with saline soaked gauze. The patient should be urgently referred to a surgeon to undergo examination and possible emergency laparotomy.

Penetrating objects

Case study 6.1 Penetrating object in situ

A teenage boy is brought to the ED by some friends. He has been in a fight and has sustained a stab wound to the right side of the upper abdomen. He is taken straight to the resuscitation room, laid on a trolley and the trauma team is summoned. The nurse who is with the patient applies O_2 15 L/min via a non-rebreathe mask and then starts to cut off the patient's clothes. The knife is still in situ, sitting under the right ribs. The patient is screaming at the nurse, saying 'take it out, take it out'. The nurse tries to reassure the patient but leaves the knife in situ. She knows this is the correct thing to do, but isn't completely sure why.

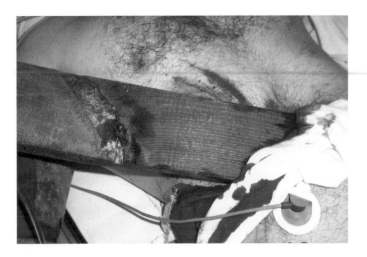

Fig. 6.2 Penetrating abdominal injury

A penetrating object to the abdomen (Figure 6.2) that is still in situ on arrival to the ED must not be removed until the patient is in an operating theatre with a surgeon present, ready to operate. The rationale for leaving the object in situ is that it may be compressing or tamponading vessels,[1] which could start to bleed uncontrollably if the object is removed. This could prove catastrophic in an uncontrolled environment.

A gunshot wound to the abdomen will normally need to be explored in surgery[6] therefore all of these types of injuries must be referred to a surgeon urgently.

PRIMARY SURVEY ASSESSMENT AND RESUSCITATION

Airway with cervical spine control

The patient's ability to maintain their own airway should be assessed first. An unconscious patient should have their airway secured with endotracheal intubation, as described in Chapter 2.

Breathing and ventilation

Signs of hypoxia such as:

- Anxiety
- Agitation
- Restlessness
- Poor oxygen saturations

May indicate that the patient who has sustained abdominal injury is in shock. Therefore, high flow oxygen, 15 L/min via a non-rebreathe mask, should be administered as a priority. *However, blunt abdominal trauma is rarely a single system injury and there may be concurrent chest problems.*

The following should be assessed to detect potential respiratory problems:

- Respiratory rate
- Chest movement, depth and effort
- External signs of chest injury, e.g. bruising or abrasions.

Abnormalities such as tachypnoea or signs of injury to the chest should be reported to a senior clinician urgently.

Circulation and haemorrhage control

Priorities for circulation and haemorrhage control in the patient with abdominal injury are broken down into three areas:

- Assessment
- Intravenous fluid therapy
- Diagnostic imaging.

Assessment

The main focus of care for the patient with abdominal trauma is to determine the source of bleeding and decide if an urgent operation is needed. This is best achieved by an experienced surgeon who should be present for all suspected or known cases of abdominal injury.

Penetrating abdominal trauma is more obvious than blunt. Patients who have sustained an injury due to blunt forces may have very subtle early signs.

Vital signs including pulse, blood pressure and level of consciousness should be recorded every 15 minutes initially to observe for signs of hypovolaemic shock. *Tachycardia is an early sign of bleeding in abdominal trauma.*

Other areas to note during assessment are:

- The patient is complaining of abdominal pain
- A reluctance to move due to the pain
- A distended or rigid abdomen
- Bruising, abrasions or wounds to the abdomen (front or back).

Intravenous fluid therapy

Intravenous access should be established and blood taken for testing and cross matching (see Chapter 2). The initiation of intravenous fluids for patients with abdominal injury remains controversial and the question of the volume and rate of fluid to be infused for the haemorrhaging patient remains to be answered definitively.[7]

A shocked, haemorrhaging patient with a systolic blood pressure of <80 will not be perfusing their organs and tissues adequately which may have devastating consequences. It seems rational therefore to give this group of patient's intravenous (IV) fluid replacement. Research into patients with penetrating torso injuries[8] suggests that limiting fluid resuscitation and having a more tolerant approach to low blood pressure may be beneficial for patient outcome. It has also been reported that IV fluids may dilute already depleted circulating blood and may cause clotting difficulties.[7,8]

National guidance suggests that IV crystalloid should be given in 250 ml portions (boli).[9] If the patient is not responding to fluids and is losing a significant amount of blood then blood transfusion should be administered.

Ultimately the patient with abdominal injury needs prompt diagnostics and a surgical consultation to determine if an operation is needed. Fluid administration should not be an alternative to this.

Diagnostic imaging

A number of diagnostic techniques are used for investigating the patient with known or suspected abdominal injury. They will help to determine if the patient needs to have an urgent operation.

1. Focused assessment with sonography for trauma (FAST)

Case study 6.2 FAST screening

A 28-year-old male patient is brought to the ED following a high speed RTA. The car he was travelling in hit a central reservation at 60 mph. The driver is critically injured and has been taken to another hospital. The patient is awake, is responding to questions and is complaining about the cervical spine collar that has been applied. His airway is clear, his respiratory rate is 25. 15 litres of oxygen are applied via a non-rebreathe mask. He has obvious injuries to his left arm, left shoulder and there is fresh bruising to the left side of his torso. His pulse is 103, his BP is 100/56 and he is in a lot of pain whilst being undressed and examined. The nurse looking after this patient reports her findings to the ED senior doctor who decides to perform a FAST. This scan shows fluid in the perisplenic region. A chest x-ray shows left lower rib fractures. He is seen immediately by an experienced surgeon to evaluate his need for surgery.

In Europe and the USA, FAST is becoming the initial investigation of choice in suspected abdominal injury.[1] The benefits of FAST include the ability to rapidly assess potential intra-abdominal bleeding and that it can be reliably carried out by

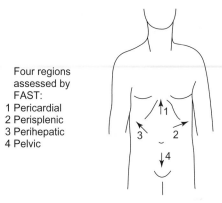

Four regions
assessed by
FAST:
1 Pericardial
2 Perisplenic
3 Perihepatic
4 Pelvic

Fig. 6.3 FAST regions

non-radiologists who have had training in the use of the machine.

FAST involves ultrasound assessment of four regions of the torso (Figure 6.3):

- The perihepatic
- The perisplenic
- The pericardial
- The pelvis.

A positive FAST result:[1]

- If bleeding is detected and the patient is cardiovascularly unstable then an immediate operation is necessary.
- If bleeding is detected and the patient is cardiovascularly stable then a CT scan may be indicated to identify where the bleeding is coming from.

2. Computerised tomography (CT)
A CT scan can provide more detailed information about intra-abdominal solid organs.[4] CT scan is only suitable for cardio-vascularly stable patients. The movement of the patient away

from the resuscitation area or operating theatre may have devastating consequences if an uncontrollable haemorrhage occurs.

3. Diagnostic peritoneal lavage (DPL)/diagnostic peritoneal aspirate (DPA)

A DPL is occasionally used to detect intra-abdominal bleeding where a FAST and CT have been inconclusive or cannot be used. Prior to the procedure a urinary catheter should be inserted to decompress the bladder and a nasogastric tube to decompress the stomach. A DPL is the technique of inserting a sterile peritoneal lavage catheter into the peritoneum, through the abdominal wall beneath the umbilicus.[6] Once in the peritoneal cavity, 10 ml/kg of warmed Hartmanns solution is infused. The fluid is then drained back out of the body (the infusion bag is placed below the level of the patient), and examined both with the naked eye and microscopically for signs of intra-abdominal haemorrhage.

A DPL is considered positive, where the patients needs an immediate surgical referral if there is:[6]

- Frank blood
- >100,000 red blood cells/ml on microscopy
- >500 white cells/ml on microscopy.

A DPA is a similar technique that may be used on the unstable patient where the FAST has been inconclusive. The procedure is the same as for a DPL, however fluid is not infused, instead the catheter is aspirated with a syringe to look for the presence of blood. Aspiration of frank blood indicates a positive DPA and the need for an immediate senior surgical referral.

Disability and dysfunction

The level of consciousness should be monitored throughout the assessment and resuscitation period to observe for signs of deterioration or worsening hypovolaemia.

The patient with a concurrent head injury should have the GCS and pupils assessed as discussed in Chapter 3.

Exposure and environmental control

It is essential that the patient with abdominal trauma is not moved excessively to reduce the risk of causing further bleeding.[10] However, the patient must be fully undressed to allow for a through examination and log rolled to ensure that posterior injuries are not missed. In penetrating abdominal injuries the buttocks, groin creases and axillae (arm pits) should be checked to ensure that wounds are not concealed in these areas. If not already considered, a urinary catheter should be inserted to monitor urine output. Additionally, a nasogastric tube may be necessary to deflate the stomach or aspirate the stomach contents prior to surgery.

CONCLUSION

Complex anatomy means that blunt abdominal injury can be difficult to detect, therefore a high index of suspicion following trauma involving the abdomen and torso must be maintained. Close monitoring of the patient's cardiovascular system and level of consciousness is essential to detect haemodynamic stability or instability. Abdominal pain and signs of hypovolaemic shock should alert the practitioner of the need for rapid expert help. Initial assessment and management of a patient with abdominal trauma focuses on recognition of the injury, timely diagnostic imaging and early intervention by a surgeon.

KEY INFORMATION BOX

- Blunt abdominal injury can be difficult to detect, therefore a high index of suspicion is needed in relation to the mechanism of injury
- Penetrating objects must be left in situ until a surgeon has assessed the injury

- All cardiovascularly unstable patients with abdominal injury need a surgical evaluation urgently
- Lower rib injuries can cause upper abdominal injuries
- Beware the patient with a reduced level of consciousness. In abdominal injury this indicates shock!
- Tachycardia associated with abdominal trauma means shock until proven otherwise
- Excessively moving patients with intra-abdominal trauma can cause further bleeding.

REFERENCES

1. Brooks A, Paynter A, Phillips E (2005) Abdominal trauma. In: Principles and practice of trauma nursing (Ed O'Shea R), 443–455. Elsevier, Edinburgh
2. Hildebrand F, Winkler M, van Griensven M, Probst C, Musahl V, Krettek C, Pape H (2006) Blunt abdominal trauma requiring laparotomy: an analysis of 342 polytraumatized patients. European Journal of Trauma 32: 430–438
3. Hodgetts T, Turner L (2006) Trauma rules 2 (2nd edn), 64–65. Blackwell Publishing, Oxford
4. Paiano R (2003) Abdominal and genitourinary trauma. In: Trauma nursing secrets (Ed Sauderson Cohen S), 85–94. Hanley & Belfus, Philadelphia
5. Demetriades D, Berne TV (2004) Chest injuries. In: Assessment and management of trauma (Eds Demetriades D, Berne TV), 27–41. LAC & USC Healthcare Network, Los Angeles
6. American College of Surgeons (2004) Abdominal trauma. In: Advanced trauma life support for doctors. Student course manual (7th edn), 131–145. American College of Surgeons, Chicago
7. Kathryn M (2006) Controversies in fluid resuscitation. Journal of Trauma Nursing 13:168–172
8. Bickell WH, Wall MJ, Pepe PE, Martin RR, Ginger VF, Allen MK, Mattox KL (1994) Immediate versus delayed fluid resuscitation for hypotensive patients with penetrat-

ing torso injuries. New England Journal of Medicine 331:1105–1109

9. National Institute for Clinical Excellence (2004) Pre-hospital initiation of fluid replacement in trauma, 28. NICE, London

10. Davies G, Lockey D (2005) Prehospital care in trauma patients. In: Critical care focus 11: Trauma (Ed Galley H), 76–83. Blackwell, Oxford

7 | Pelvic Injuries

Elaine Cole

Pelvic fractures occur in 20% of multiple trauma cases, with a mortality rate of 10–30%, increased in open or compound fractures.[1] The significant morbidity and mortality seen in pelvic trauma are due to pelvic artery haemorrhage and associated intra-abdominal bleeding.[2] Pelvic fractures may result from low impact forces such as a trip or fall, or high impact forces such as a high speed road traffic accident (RTA). Low impact, low energy mechanisms can cause stable pelvic fractures, which can be treated conservatively, i.e. without operative intervention. High impact, high energy mechanisms can cause unstable pelvic fractures with associated severe bleeding that can be life threatening. Assessment and early management of pelvic injuries focuses on recognition of haemodynamic instability and accessing expert help urgently to control haemorrhage.

The aim of this chapter is to understand the principles of rapid assessment, resuscitation and stabilisation of the person with a pelvic injury.

LEARNING OBJECTIVES
By the end of this chapter the reader will be able to:

❏ Describe the anatomy of the pelvis
❏ Identify the mechanisms of injury that cause pelvic fractures
❏ Understand the classification of pelvic fractures
❏ Describe assessment and management priorities in relation to ABCDE.

ANATOMY OF THE PELVIS

The bony pelvis is the bridge between the spine and the lower extremities.[2] Essentially the pelvis is made up of three bones – the sacrum and the two innominate bones (Figure 7.1). These three bones are attached by three joints:

- The two sacroiliac (SI) joints posteriorly (at the back)
- The symphysis pubis anteriorly (at the front).

Strong ligaments, such as the anterior and posterior sacro-iliac ligaments, provide support and structure to the bony pelvis, allowing it to bear much of the body's weight. If the pelvic ligaments are disrupted and the joints of the pelvis become widened, the structure of the pelvis can become unstable.

There is a rich arterial blood supply to the pelvis. The main iliac arteries are situated within the bony pelvic ring including:

- The common iliac
- The internal iliac
- The deep circumflex iliac
- The external iliac.

Fractures of the pelvic bones or widening of the SI joints can injure the iliac vessels and severe bleeding can result.

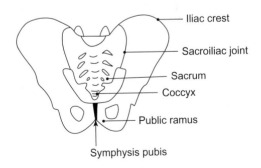

Iliac crest

Sacroiliac joint

Sacrum

Coccyx

Public ramus

Symphysis pubis

Fig. 7.1 The pelvis

Situated within or near to the pelvis are a number of structures, which if damaged during a traumatic injury can cause infection. Additionally, long term functional problems can occur if these injuries are not detected and treated appropriately. These structures include:

- The bladder
- The urethra
- The prostate gland (in males)
- The female reproductive organs
- The sigmoid colon and rectum.

MECHANISM OF PELVIC INJURY

Case study 7.1 Pelvic injury

A 55-year-old male cyclist has been involved in an RTA with a heavy goods vehicle. The patient was hit on the right hand side and thrown from his bicycle.

Paramedics report that the patient is complaining of right hip pain and thigh pain. They are concerned that he may have an unstable injury. When they undressed the patient at scene to examine him, they noted a large abrasion over the right iliac crest and that the pelvis looks deformed – 'flatter on the right side in comparison to the left'. A pelvic binder has been applied at scene.

His vital signs at scene show that the patient is haemodynamically compromised:

RR 24, HR 112, BP 134/90, GCS 14 (slightly confused).

Pelvic injuries are usually caused by blunt force. When unstable fractures and posterior ligament disruption are present, this suggests that a major force was involved.[3]

Significant (i.e. severe and possibly unstable) pelvic fractures result from:

- Road traffic accidents
- Motorcycle accidents

- Pedestrian vs. vehicle collision
- Cyclist vs. vehicle collision
- Falls from a great height.

The major force that is responsible for causing a significant pelvic fracture often causes other injuries[3,4] and the incidence of associated abdominal injuries is high in all age groups.[5]

Other injuries include:

- Intra-abdominal injuries resulting in peritoneal and retro-peritoneal haemorrhage
- Injury to vascular structures within the abdomen
- Injury to the thoracic aorta.

All of these injuries can cause the patient to become profoundly hypovolaemic, which may be life threatening if not detected and treated urgently. Recognition of haemodynamic instability and timely FAST scanning are essential during the assessment process.

Four patterns of force are generally seen relating mechanism of injury to classification of pelvic fracture.

CLASSIFICATION OF PELVIC FRACTURES

Young and Burgess[6] and Tile[7] are two of the main classification systems used for describing pelvic fractures. Whilst both systems differ slightly, they can be broadly divided into four classifications of injury. The direction and type of force that has impacted on the patient causes the resulting injury (Table 7.1).

Anterior-posterior (AP) compression fractures (Figure 7.2)

The force associated with AP compression fractures may cause a disruption to the symphysis pubis joint. If this joint is disrupted (or widened) >2.5 cm,[2] then there is a risk of instability to the pelvis, especially if posterior ligaments have been injured.[2,3] This type of injury is sometimes called an 'open book fracture' due to the widening of the pelvic ring. Disruption of the SI joints may also occur suggesting injury to the iliac vessels and therefore haemorrhage.

Table 7.1 Force relating to pelvic injury classification

Force	Injury classification
Force (compression) is applied to the front of the pelvis (anterior) or back (posterior) or both (anterior-posterior or posterior-anterior)	Anterior-posterior compression injury
Force is applied to one side (unilateral) or both sides (bilateral) of the pelvic ring	Lateral compression injury
High energy force is applied vertically, from foot to head or head to foot, shearing one side of the pelvis (the hemi-pelvis) away from the pelvic ring	Vertical shear injury

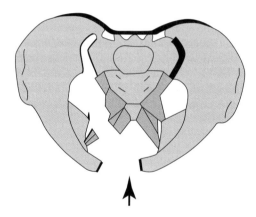

Fig. 7.2 Anterior-posterior pelvic injury. (Permission from K Brohi. Source www.trauma.org)

Lateral compression injury (Figure 7.3)

A force or impact from the side is associated with lateral compression fractures. The force causes internal rotation or compression of one side (or both) of the hemi-pelvis.[1,3] *Care must be taken to avoid log rolling the patient onto the affected side if at all possible, as this can worsen the injury.*

This type of pelvic injury may cause displaced fractures of the pubic bone and there is a risk of bone causing structural

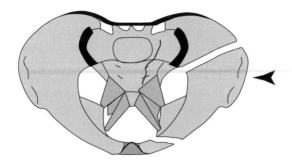

Fig. 7.3 Lateral compression pelvic injury. (Permission from K Brohi. Source www.trauma.org)

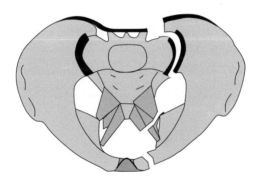

Fig. 7.4 Vertical shear pelvic injury. (Permission from K Brohi. Source www. trauma.org)

damage to the underlying organs such as the bladder, urethra and uterus.

Vertical shear injury (Figure 7.4)

The high energy shearing force associated with this injury causes major disruption to the bony ring, the SI joints, stabilising ligaments and iliac vessels. This leads to major pelvic instability and life-threatening haemorrhage.[4,8] This type of injury may produce significant damage to the internal pelvic organs, producing rectal, urethral and vaginal bleeding.

Complex pattern injury

The fourth classification of injury relates to a combination of two or more fracture types described above, sometimes known as complex pattern pelvic injury.[2-4]

Open or compound pelvic fractures

Open pelvic fractures are defined as a bony injury with associated skin or tissue loss. This can be as simple as a laceration to the skin to a full degloving injury where skin, subcutaneous fat and muscle are damaged.[4] The perineum, rectum and vagina should be inspected to ensure wounds in these areas are not missed. The risk of mortality increases with an open pelvic fracture due to haemorrhage, clotting problems and infection (from external contamination and bowel/bladder contamination).

PRIMARY SURVEY ASSESSMENT AND RESUSCITATION

Case study 7.2 Analgesia for major injury

A 34-year-old motor scooter driver has lost control of her vehicle in an RTA and has ended up beneath another vehicle.

On arrival to the ED she is conscious, very distressed, crying out in pain. The paramedics have administered inhaled nitrous oxide (Entonox) to the patient with little effect.

She is extremely upset due to the pain and is finding it hard to lie still on the trolley. A cannula is inserted into her left arm and 5 mg/5 ml of morphine sulphate is administered intravenously (10 mg morphine sulphate mixed with 10 ml normal saline to produce 1 mg per ml).

50 mg cyclizine is also administered to prevent nausea. After 5 minutes the pain is reassessed. The patient is calmer

---

> and states that the pain is less but still present. A further
> 3 mg/3 ml of morphine sulphate are administered with
> good effect.

In the conscious patient with a pelvic injury, the need for
analgesia should be determined early. This should not detract
from the systematic ABCDE assessment, however injury to
the bony pelvis can be excruciatingly painful. Intravenous
opiates such as morphine should be prescribed and administered, with an antiemetic to prevent associated nausea and
vomiting.

Airway with cervical spine control
As for all traumatic injury, the patient's ability to maintain
their airway should be assessed. Significant hypovolaemia
and the resulting hypoxia may cause the patient's level of
consciousness to deteriorate, causing airway compromise.
The airway should be assessed and managed systematically
as described in Chapter 2.

The cervical spine should be immobilised. A significant
pelvic fracture is caused by a major force, therefore the risk of
an associated spinal injury is high.

Breathing and ventilation
Assessment of breathing and ventilation should include:

- Respiratory rate
- Respiratory effort and depth
- Oxygen saturation monitoring
- Assessment of chest wall to look for signs of injury, bruis-
  ing, abrasions.

Abnormalities in breathing and ventilation should be reported
to a senior clinician as they may imply a concurrent thoracic
injury. Tachypnoea (a high respiratory rate) may be an early

indicator of hypovolaemic shock. Hypovolaemia caused by pelvic injuries will result in hypoxia, therefore all patients with suspected pelvic injuries should have high flow oxygen administered, 15 L/min via a non-rebreathe mask.

Circulation and haemorrhage control

The circulatory assessment of a patient with a pelvic injury should focus on recognition of haemodynamic instability and prompt intervention, to prevent the patient deteriorating into hypovolaemic shock. Substantial haemorrhage can occur with pelvic fractures, especially when there is disruption of the bony pelvic ring.[1] Concurrent abdominal injuries or fractures of the femurs can increase the risk of haemorrhage significantly. Where the mechanism of injury is suggestive of a pelvic injury, close observation of the following vital signs is essential:

- Heart rate
- Blood pressure
- Capillary refill time
- Level of consciousness.

Other signs and symptoms of a pelvic injury include:

- Pelvic pain
- Pelvic deformity or asymmetry
- Bruising to the scrotum, buttocks, perineum or flank
- Haematuria
- Blood from the external urethral meatus
- Pain over the symphysis pubis
- Lower back, hip or lower abdominal pain
- A haemodynamically 'shocked' patient.

Non-invasive stabilisation should be applied, such as a pelvic splint, pelvic binder or a sheet tied around the pelvis.[9] This holds tissue and bone in place and allows a blood clot to form.

Two large bore venous cannulae should be inserted and trauma blood tests taken (see Chapter 2). In addition, blood should be taken for group and cross matching in readiness for the patient requiring blood transfusion. If the patient has sustained an unstable pelvic injury and is losing blood, intravenous fluids should be administered. The anatomy of the pelvis means that the risk of arterial haemorrhage is significant, therefore:

If the patient is losing blood, this needs to be replaced by blood and clotting factors as soon as possible.

Infusing large amounts of crystalloid will only replace intravenous volume and will not enhance oxygen delivery or clotting ability, therefore a blood transfusion is necessary. The universal donor, O negative blood, may have to be administered if fully cross-matched blood is unavailable in the early stages of care. Patients are at risk of developing problems with clotting (coagulopathy) following severe traumatic injury[2] therefore baseline clotting blood tests should be taken.

Once a bladder injury has been excluded placement of a urinary catheter may be beneficial to help monitor fluid balance and the efficacy of fluid resuscitation. The following may indicate injury to the bladder/urethra:[3]

- A lateral compression injury (where bone is displaced inwards)
- Bleeding from the external urethral meatus
- A high-riding prostate gland (detected on rectal examination in male patients).

On trying to pass a urinary catheter, if resistance or difficulty is encountered it is advisable to stop and seek senior help.

Disability and dysfunction

The patient's level of consciousness should be monitored as a deterioration may indicate haemodynamic instability due to hypovolaemic shock. If a concurrent head injury is present, the level of consciousness should be assessed using the Glasgow Coma Scale.

Exposure and environmental control

The patient should be fully undressed, including the underwear, to allow for a thorough assessment and examination. Wounds to the pelvic region should be reported, as they may be indicative of an open pelvic injury.

The patient will need to be log rolled to allow for the posterior surface to be examined. The clinician examining the patient will perform a rectal examination to check for bony fragments from the pelvis that may have penetrated the bowel. Female patients should have a vaginal examination performed to rule out injury to the vagina, cervix or uterus.[4]

The log roll should be carried out with extreme care, minimising excess movement to the injured pelvis. *Multiple log rolls and unnecessary movement should be avoided to minimise the risk of causing further pelvic instability and increasing haemorrhage.*

MANAGEMENT OF PELVIC INJURIES

Once the patient assessment has been completed and a pelvic fracture is suspected, a number of interventions may be necessary. An experienced clinician should carefully examine the pelvis to decide if the injury has caused mechanical instability.[3] This means a gentle manipulation of the pelvis, feeling for movement or deformity rather than vigorous springing which should be avoided. Definitive management of the injury will be determined by the patient's haemodynamic status and the assessment findings (Figure 7.5).[10]

Diagnostic imaging

X-ray

In most EDs the first line diagnostic imaging will be a plain x-ray which will help to determine the type and severity of the pelvic fracture.

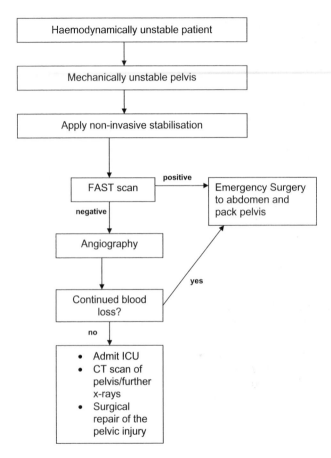

Fig. 7.5 Decision making algorithm for the management of pelvic fractures.[10]

Focused Assessment with Sonography in Trauma (FAST)

All patients with pelvic injuries should have a FAST scan to detect pelvic or lower abdominal bleeding.[11] This may have to be repeated if the patient continues to be haemodynamically unstable to ensure that intra-abdominal injury has not been missed.

Genitourinary tract evaluation

A cystogram or urethrogram may be necessary to look for urethral or bladder injury. Many of these injuries are missed in the early stages of care.[4] However, this type of imaging should not take priority over the need to resuscitate the patient and control haemorrhage.

CT scanning

For the haemodynaically stable patient, a CT scan of the pelvis may be requested for more detailed information about the pelvic injury.[4] It is not safe to send a haemodynamically unstable patient to the CT scan. Alternative intervention may be necessary in this scenario, such as angiography and embolisation.

Haemorrhage control

If the patient is continuing to lose blood and is haemodynamically unstable, the priority is to stop the bleeding within the pelvis. This can be achieved by:

- External fixation
- Angiography and embolisation
- Surgery.

External fixation

External fixation of the pelvic bones is an application of metal frames and clamps in an attempt to restore the bony ring to its normal anatomical position, tamponade (or compress) the bleeding and decrease haemorrhage.[4] It is not effective in cases of arterial bleeding and is not suitable for all fracture types, being used predominantly for anterior-poster fractures.[12]

Angiography and embolisation

Angiography is used for definitive diagnosis of pelvic vascular injuries.[13] Pelvic angiography assists in the identification of arterial bleeding sites that may need embolisation, in order to control the haemorrhage associated with pelvic fractures.[10,13] The procedure is carried out in an x-ray suite and resuscitation equipment must be available because of the unstable nature of the patient with a pelvic haemorrhage.

Surgery

The decision to take the patient for surgery will be made by a senior clinician based on:[4,10]

- If there is ongoing blood loss (the patient continues to be unstable) and the pelvis needs to be packed
- If the patient requires abdominal surgery based on the FAST scan findings – abdominal packing
- If the patient needs urgent surgery to intra-pelvic organs, e.g. an emergency colostomy for a bowel injury
- If the pelvic fracture needs open reduction and fixation (ORIF) – although this is usually done at a later stage once the patient is stable.

CONCLUSION

Fractures of the pelvis are caused by blunt trauma, and a severe injury suggests that major force was involved. The risk of other injuries, in areas such as the abdomen or thorax, is high, and therefore the patient needs careful assessment and examination. Morbidity and mortality rates increase with severe pelvic injuries, due to associated haemorrhage, therefore close assessment of the patient's haemodynamic status is essential. Early recognition of patients with active bleeding is vital to ensure that haemorrhage control can be carried out in a timely manner.

KEY INFORMATION BOX

- Patients with pelvic injuries need early, effective analgesia
- Tachycardia, tachypnoea and an altered level of consciousness are all indicators of haemorrhage

---

- The risk of associated abdominal and thoracic injury means that a FAST scan should always be performed
- Minimise movement of the patient with a pelvic injury to minimise further bleeding
- Haemodynamically unstable patients with severe pelvic injuries need blood and clotting products transfused rather than crystalloids
- The CT scanner is an unsafe environment for the haemodynamically unstable patient.

REFERENCES

1. Smith M (2005) Orthopaedic trauma. In: Principles and practice of trauma nursing (Ed O'Shea R), 379–419. Elsevier, Edinburgh

2. Thornton DD (2002) Pelvic ring fractures. http://www.emedicine.com/radio/topic546.htm

3. American College of Surgeons (2004) Abdominal trauma. In: Advanced trauma life support for doctors. Student course manual (7th edn), 131–145. American College of Surgeons, Chicago

4. Prayson MJ, Gruen GS (2002) Pelvic fractures. In: The trauma manual (2nd edn) (Eds Peitzman AB, Rhodes M, Schwab CW, Yealy DM, Fabian TDC), 311–318. Lippincott, Williams & Wilkins, Philadelphia

5. Demetriades D, Karaiskakis M, Velmahos GC, Alo K, Murray J, Chan L (2003) Pelvic fractures in pediatric and adult trauma patients: are they different injuries? Journal of Trauma, Injury Infection & Critical Care 54: 1146–1151

6. Young JW, Burgess AR, Brumback RJ, Poka A (1986) Pelvic fractures: value of plain radiography in early assessment and management. Radiology 160:445–451

7. Tile M (1988) Pelvic ring fractures: should they be fixed? Journal of Bone and Joint Surgery 70:1–12

8. Routt ML, Nork SE, Mills WJ (2002) High energy pelvic ring disruptions. Orthopaedic Clinics of North America 33:59–72

9. Hodgetts T, Turner L (2006). Trauma rules 2 (2nd Edn), 118–119. Blackwell Publishing, Oxford

10. Brohi K (2000) Haemodynamic Instability associated with pelvic fracture. http://160.129.198.247/ota/s2k/algo/kbroal.htm

11. Brohi K (2000) Focused Assessment with Sonography for Trauma (FAST). http://www.trauma.org/index.php/main/article/214/

12. Tucker MC, Nork SE, Simonian PT, Routt C (2000) Simple anterior pelvic external fixation. Journal of Trauma, Injury Infection & Critical Care 49:989–994

13. Federle MP (2002) Imaging of trauma patients. In: The trauma manual (2nd edn) (Eds Peitzman AB, Rhodes M, Schwab CW, Yealy DM, Fabian TC), 109–118. Lippincott, Williams & Wilkins, Philadelphia

8 | Extremity Trauma

Elaine Cole

Extremity trauma, such as fractures or crush injury to the limbs, is commonly associated with major trauma following blunt injury. Whilst extremity trauma is rarely life threatening, severe injuries such as degloving, partial amputations or compartment syndrome are certainly limb threatening. Limb injury in the survivors of major trauma is a common source of disability affecting the patient's return to their pre-injury state.[1]

Some extremity trauma is very subtle and may not be detected during the initial assessment of the patient.[2] Injuries to the scaphoid bone or a growth plate fracture in a child can easily be missed, especially if the patient is unconscious or intubated and therefore unable to complain of pain or dysfunction.

Extremity trauma can be visually distracting. There is a risk that an injury such as a traumatic amputation or a mangled extremity can distract the team from assessment of life-threatening injuries. Considering this, a systematic approach to assessment continues to be the priority with extremity trauma, dealing with extremity injuries in 'C', 'E' or in the secondary phase of assessment as the injury severity dictates.

The aim of this chapter is to understand the principles of rapid assessment, resuscitation and stabilisation of the person with an extremity injury.

LEARNING OBJECTIVES
By the end of this chapter the reader will be able to:

❏ Define life-threatening extremity injuries and recognise signs and symptoms

❑ Define limb-threatening extremity injury and recognise signs and symptoms
❑ Understand compartment syndrome and how to identify it
❑ Identify complications of crush injury
❑ Describe assessment and management priorities in relation to ABCDE.

LIFE- AND LIMB-THREATENING EXTREMITY TRAUMA

Many structures may be involved in extremity trauma, such as bones, nerves, blood vessels, skin or a combination of the above. The assessment and examination of limbs may not occur until other major problems have been ruled out or treated, however Table 8.1 shows a list of life- and limb-threatening injuries that should be considered in any patient with extremity trauma.

Bony injuries

Fractures and dislocations occur in a significant number of trauma patients.[2] The mechanism of injury usually involves blunt force, however a penetrating force such as a bullet or high speed missile can fracture a bone. Bony injury can be broken down into a number of categories, dependent on the structures involved.

Dislocation

A dislocation is where there is a complete loss of congruity (or connection) between the two bones in a joint.[3] Commonly it is seen in the shoulder, however a dislocation can occur in any joint, such as the elbow, the hip, the knee. Injury to the stabilising ligaments around the joint can occur, and if the joint is not realigned or *relocated* in a timely manner, there may be resulting injury to the nerves and vessels distal (away from) to the injury.

Features of a dislocation include:

• Pain
• Reduction in movement

Table 8.1 Life- and limb-threatening extremity trauma

Injury	Presenting features	Life or limb threatening
Fractured femur	Swelling, deformity and pain to the affected thigh Hypovolaemic shock	Life threatening due to haemorrhage risk
Open fracture	Wound above fracture site Bone visible through wound Damaged or devitalised tissue Possible associated haemorrhage	Life threatening due to haemorrhage risk Later risk to life from sepsis and fat embolism
Dislocation or displaced fracture	Deformity, swelling, pain, reduction in movement Possible neurovascular deficit if nerves or vessels are involved	Limb threatening due to motor function problems if limb not realigned Potential vascular and/or compromise
Traumatic amputation	Partial or complete loss of limb Possible associated haemorrhage Damaged or devitalised tissue	Limb threatening due to loss of limb Life threatening due to haemorrhage risk. Later risk to life from sepsis
Wound with arterial involvement	Fresh red blood spurting from the wound Hypovolaemic shock	Life threatening due to haemorrhage risk
Severe crush injury	Swollen painful limb Massive tissue loss or degloving injury Associated haemorrhage (internal or external) Associated neurovascular damage	Life threatening due to haemorrhage risk, sepsis, clotting problems Limb threatening due to compartment syndrome or the need for an amputation
Compartment syndrome	Severe pain Loss of sensation or movement Swollen, tense limb Associated with fractures and crush injuries	Limb threatening
Vascular injury	Distal neurovascular deficit: pallor, pain, paralysis, paraesthesia and cool temperature	Limb threatening due to vascular compromise
Nerve injury	Reduction or loss of sensation Reduction or loss of movement	Limb threatening

- Deformity at the affected joint
- Shortening of the limb.

Dislocations should be relocated as soon as possible. This should occur once life-threatening injuries have been ruled out or treated. However, simultaneous management of orthopaedic injuries may occur during a trauma-team resuscitation.

Subluxation

Subluxation refers to the partial loss of congruity (or connection) between two bones in a joint.[3] The capsules around the joint and the supporting ligaments are undamaged and remain in place. Whilst this is not a significant injury, the risk of a subluxation becoming a full dislocation should be considered.

Fracture

A fracture can be defined as a break in the continuity of a bone.[4] The severity of a fracture can vary greatly depending on where the injury is (a finger compared to a femur, for example), and the type of fracture that has been sustained.

Features of a fracture include:

- Pain
- Deformity (if the bones have moved out of normal alignment)
- Swelling, due to surrounding soft tissue injury and bleeding
- Reduction in function
- Shortening of the limb (in a hip fracture for example).

Fractures can be divided into two groups:

- Open (or also known as compound) – where the bone is exposed to the external environment through a wound
- Closed – where the skin is intact.

Following assessment, examination and x-ray (covered later in this chapter) the fracture can be further classified according to:

- Fracture type – for example transverse, oblique, greenstick
- Morphology – simple (in two parts) or comminuted (in many parts)
- Location – proximal (nearest), middle or distal (furthest away)
- Position – undisplaced, displaced, angulated, rotated, etc.

The classification and severity of the fracture will determine if emergency orthopaedic intervention is necessary. Two types of fractures have significance for the major trauma patient – open fractures and fractures of the femoral shaft.

Open fractures

An open fracture (or compound fracture) means that the bone is exposed to the external environment through a wound in the skin surface. They are significant injuries,[2,3] as muscle and skin as well as bone have been injured. A large amount of skin or soft tissue injury above a fracture poses a large infection risk. Early wound irrigation and splinting are essential. Urgent referral to an orthopaedic surgeon must be made as the injury may need fixation and debridement. Intravenous antibiotics and tetanus toxoid prophylaxis are necessary in the majority of cases.

To minimise the risk of further contamination and infection, a photograph should be taken of the wound then a secure dressing applied until the surgeon is ready to treat the wound and the fracture.

Femoral fractures

Considerable force is required to fracture the shaft of the femur[4] and associated injuries are common, such as pelvic fractures or hip injury. The femur is a large bone, and injury to the shaft can result in a large volume haemorrhage, typically 1.5–2 litres per femur.[2,4] Open or compound fractures of the femur can result in exsanguinating haemorrhage.

Features of a femoral shaft fracture include:

- Pain
- Swelling
- Deformity
- Muscle spasm
- Shortening
- Signs of hypovolaemic shock (tachycardia, altered level of consciousness, etc.).

This is a very painful injury, therefore in the conscious patient intravenous opioid analgesia such as morphine, or a femoral nerve block is essential. Immobilisation of the fracture using a splint such as a Donway splint™, a Sager splint™ or a Thomas splint will help to reduce pain and potential haemorrhage. Urgent orthopaedic referral is necessary for definitive management.

Traumatic amputation

Traumatic amputations (Figures 8.1, 8.2) are true life- and limb-threatening injuries.[3] They are devastating for the patient, physically and psychologically. Amputations can be caused by RTAs (vehicle occupants, pedestrian or cyclist vs. vehicle), industrial incidents, agricultural incidents or explosions. Haemorrhage may occur due to damaged vessels and therefore the patient should be monitored for hypovolaemic shock.[1] If the remaining part of the limb or digit is bleeding, a sterile covering should be applied, direct pressure and elevation instigated.

Re-implantation of the amputated part may be possible depending on the severity of injury to the body part and the status of the patient. The amputated body part should be carefully wrapped in wet gauze and placed in a plastic bag or plastic container. This should then be placed in an ice bath (water and ice mix). *Never place the amputated body part directly onto ice as it will freeze and cause frostbite.*[1–3]

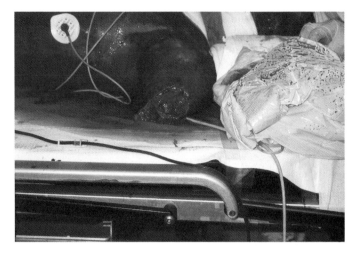

Fig. 8.1 Traumatic amputation of the left arm

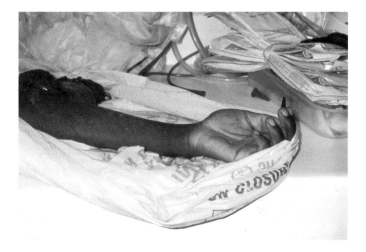

Fig. 8.2 Amputated arm

Partial amputations may result in the limb or digit still being attached to some extent. Often the skin, tissue and bone are severely damaged or mangled[3,4] and may need to be amputated. The remaining tissue should be covered with a sterile dressing until expert advice is available.

Wounds

Injury to the skin, subcutaneous tissue, muscles and tendons can be caused by blunt or penetrating trauma.[5]

Blunt trauma causes:

- Shearing (or tearing) of tissue
- Crush injuries where there is often widespread damaged tissue with a high infection risk.

Penetrating trauma causes:

- Knife wounds, impalement wounds where minimal tissue damage results
- Gunshot wounds (especially high velocity) where large amounts of soft tissue injury may result.

Whilst some wounds may appear to be innocuous, all are at risk of infection due to foreign material contamination. Once the assessment has been completed, all wounds should be thoroughly irrigated as soon as possible, rather than relying on antibiotics and surgery. This is best achieved by delivering normal saline directly from the end of a giving set connected to the fluid bag.[6]

The solution to pollution is dilution![6]

Extensive wounds can cause severe haemorrhage, over-whelming infection, and loss of function due to nerve damage or ischaemia.[5] Where the skin and underlying soft tissue have been injured and peeled back over the bones, this is called a degloving injury (Figure 8.3).[4] A senior clinician should review all significant soft tissue injuries, as surgical debridement of devitalised tissue and exploration of underlying structures will be necessary.

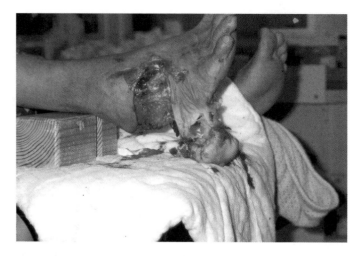

Fig. 8.3 Degloving injury of the foot

Case study 8.1 Tetanus toxoid immunisation

A 78-year-old man is brought to the ED following a fall from a ladder in his garden. Following ABCDE assessment he is diagnosed with a right-sided fractured femur, a right wrist injury and a large tear in the skin of his right upper arm.

The nurse looking after Mr Martin enquires about his tetanus immunisation status. He remembers having a tetanus injection in the army in the 1950s and a 'booster' following a hand wound 'over twenty years ago'. As it is uncertain if he has life long immunity a course of tetanus toxoid injection is started as per Department of Health advice (see Chapter 2).

In any wound the skin has been breached therefore the patient's tetanus immunity should be established. A tetanus toxoid booster may be required, however a large area of devitalised skin and tissue is considered a tetanus prone wound and tetanus immunoglobulin may be necessary.[7]

Crush injuries

Crush injuries can cause extensive underlying damage. If muscle is severely injured, muscle protein (myoglobin) is released into the systemic circulation.[2] Myoglobin is then filtered in the kidneys, causing damage to the glomerular filtration system. This can cause acute renal failure, resulting in rhabdomyolysis, dark urine containing blood. Senior clinical advice should be sought, as intravenous fluid therapy and maintaining a greater than normal urine output is necessary.

Compartment syndrome

Compartment syndrome occurs when there is increased pressure within the limited space of a muscle compartment. This causes reduced blood flow to the tissues below the level of the injury. Compartment syndrome of the leg, arm or thigh should be considered in trauma patients who have sustained significant orthopaedic or vascular injuries.[8] If left untreated or unrecognised, compartment syndrome can cause irreversible necrosis and permanent loss of function to the affected limb.

Case study 8.2 Compartment syndrome

A 40-year-old woman has an open comminuted fracture of her left tibia and fibula following an RTA (she was a pedestrian hit by a car). She is in the ED awaiting emergency surgery for exploration under anaesthetic and possible open reduction and fixation of the injury. She has a lower leg splint in situ and her leg is elevated on a pillow. Prior to the splint application she was given 5 mg morphine and 50 mg cyclizine intravenously.

Half an hour after the analgesia has been administered, the patient starts to complain of pain in her left leg, and tingling in her left foot. The nurse looking after her checks

---

that the splint is not too tight and then administers a further 5 mg of morphine as prescribed. Despite this, the patient continues to complain of severe leg pain and numbness in her foot. Pedal pulses in the foot are present and she is reluctant to wiggle her toes due to the pain. A senior doctor is called, as the nurse is worried that the patient is developing compartment syndrome.

It is difficult to diagnose compartment syndrome as the signs and symptoms can develop slowly, and may not appear obvious until the increased pressure has become critical. Evidence of the '6 P's'[9] in a high risk patient (Box 8.1) should alert the practitioner to the possibility of compartment syndrome developing:

- Pain (severe)
- Pressure (swollen tense limb)
- Paraesthesia (loss of sensation)
- Paralysis (loss of movement)
- Pallor (a late sign)
- Pulses (present until the very late stages when pressure is very high).

The unconscious patient will not complain of pain or other early signs. Therefore if compartment syndrome is suspected, expert help should be sought (orthopaedic, vascular or plastic surgery) to measure compartment pressures. Normal

---

Box 8.1 Injuries at risk of developing compartment syndrome

- Severe crush injuries
- Vascular injuries
- Fractures
- Severe contusions
- A swollen limb beneath a cast or splint

---

compartment pressure is <10 mmHg.[8] Pressure over 30 mmHg suggests that compartment syndrome is present and that treatment is required. Treatment is based on returning the compartment pressures to normal[8] and involves a surgical fasciotomy where an incision is made releasing the muscle compartments in the affected limb.

Vascular injury

Vascular injuries are caused by both penetrating and blunt trauma:[2,10]

- Vascular injury can be limb threatening if not promptly recognised and treated
- Arterial injury is particularly significant as muscle does not tolerate a lack of arterial blood flow for longer than 6 hours before necrosis occurs.

Signs of a vascular injury are divided into *hard* and *soft* (Table 8.2).[10,11] On recognition of the signs the following should be considered:

- Where hard signs are present, senior expert help must be sought immediately.
- If there is a constriction to the vascular blood flow in the limb, such as a tight splint or dressing, this must be loosened immediately.

Table 8.2 Signs of arterial or vascular injury

Hard signs: patient needs urgent surgery	Soft signs: patient can be observed and affected area further explored
Absent or diminished pulses in the affected limb	Wound or injury near to an artery
Severe active bleeding	Small non-pulsatile haematoma
Pulsatile, expanding haematoma	Minor bleeding/history of bleeding
Bruit or thrill (unusual sounds made as blood passes through an obstruction, heard using a stethoscope)	
Pallor and coolness in the limb	

- Fractures or dislocations, which may be compromising vascular blood flow, should be relocated and stabilised as soon as possible.
- Ongoing monitoring of pulses in the affected limb must be carried out whilst waiting for expert help.

Doppler ultrasound may be carried out to measure the speed and direction of blood in the vessels. Angiography may be required to establish the site of the injury and surgical repair may be necessary.[11]

Nerve injury

Peripheral nerves may be damaged by blunt or penetrating trauma. A nerve may be completely severed by a knife or impaling object. More commonly, nerves can be compressed or stretched by a fractured bone or swollen tissue following blunt injury. Signs and symptoms suggestive of a nerve injury include:

- Reduction or loss of motor power (movement and strength)
- Reduction or loss of sensory function (ability to feel sharp and light touch)
- Paraesthesia (numbness or tingling).

It is difficult to properly assess peripheral nerve function in a multiply injured patient with distracting injuries or an altered level of consciousness. Nerve assessment may need to be repeated in the definitive care setting or after the patient has been stabilised.[2]

Nerve injuries can be classified into three groups:[4,12]

- *Neuropraxia:* Usually due to blunt trauma, nerves are intact but 'concussed' or bruised, prognosis for recovery is very good.
- *Axonotemesis:* Usually due to a crush or stretch injury, some division of nerve fibres (the axons) but the nerve sheath is intact, good prognosis for recovery.

- *Neurotmesis:* Usually due to penetrating injury or severe blunt force, involves a severed nerve and nerve sheath, needs surgical repair.

PRIMARY SURVEY ASSESSMENT AND RESUSCITATION

Airway with cervical spine control
As for all trauma patients, assessment of the airway with simultaneous cervical spine control is the first priority for the patient with an extremity injury. Extremity injury can be distracting in its appearance, therefore it is important to focus on the ABCDE assessment priorities.

Breathing and ventilation
Assessment of breathing and ventilation should include:

- Respiratory rate
- Respiratory effort and depth
- Oxygen saturation monitoring.

Tachypnoea (a high respiratory rate) may be an early indicator of hypovolaemic shock. Hypovolaemia due to femoral shaft fractures or arterial injury will result in hypoxia, therefore all patients suspected of having such injuries should have high flow oxygen administered, 15 L/min via a non-rebreathe mask.

Circulation and haemorrhage control
The circulatory assessment of a patient with an extremity injury should focus on recognition of haemodynamic instability and prompt intervention, to prevent the patient deteriorating into hypovolaemic shock. Substantial haemorrhage can occur with femoral fractures, traumatic amputations and vascular injuries.[2,3] Where either type of injury is suspected, close observation of the following vital signs is essential:

- Heart rate
- Blood pressure

- Capillary refill time
- Level of consciousness.

Two large bore venous cannulae should be inserted and trauma blood tests taken (see Chapter 2). In addition, blood should be taken for group and cross matching in readiness for the patient requiring blood transfusion.

If the patient is losing blood due to a significant extremity injury, this needs to be replaced as soon as possible.

External haemorrhage control

Whether from an open wound, amputated limb or vascular injury, external haemorrhage should have:

- Direct pressure applied
- The limb elevated.

In cases of major arterial bleeding a tourniquet may be used *under the supervision of senior expert help*.[2] This should be used judiciously as prolonged application of a tourniquet can cause neurovascular injury.

Splinting limb injuries

Application of splinting may be beneficial in helping to realign fractures and reduce associated blood loss. Temporary splinting has a number of benefits whilst the patient is in the ED:[1]

- Reduction in haemorrhage
- Prevention of further tissue damage
- Help to reduce pain by reducing movement of the affected area
- Reduce the incidence of fat embolism.

Application of a splint can be very painful for the patient, therefore adequate analgesia such as intravenous morphine, or a nerve block, should be administered prior to the procedure.

Splintage can cause increased pressure to the affected area if applied too tightly, therefore splints should be checked regularly and the neurovascular status of the distal end of the limb assessed, specifically for:

- Skin colour
- Skin temperature
- Sensation
- Pedal pulses.

Disability and dysfunction

The patient's level of consciousness should be monitored as a deterioration may indicate haemodynamic instability due to hypovolaemia. If a concurrent head injury is present, the level of consciousness should be assessed using the Glasgow Coma Scale.

Exposure and environmental control

The patient should be fully undressed, including the underwear, to allow for a thorough assessment and examination.

Limb injury is a common source of disability affecting the patient's return to their pre-injury state,[1] however some extremity trauma is very subtle and may not be detected during the initial assessment and management of the patient.[2] The need to identify and treat life-threatening injuries may take priority over the assessment and examination of extremities, and this may be carried out at a later stage in the patient's care.

If limbs are not formally assessed in the ED then this should be clearly documented in the patient's notes to ensure that it is carried out in the definitive care setting.

Limb assessment

Assessment and examination of the limbs should be systematic and include the following:[1]

- Look – for deformity, swelling, shortening of the limb, skin colour, bruising, wounds
- Feel – for pain or tenderness, crepitus, pulses, temperature, sensation

- Move – to assess the range of active and passive movement and power, joint stability (assessment of movement needs to be carried out by an experienced practitioner with the appropriate training).

Following the assessment and examination, x-rays of limbs, bones or joints may be requested if bony injury is suspected. Again this may be carried out at a later stage of the patient's care if other injuries are the priority.

If an extremity injury is diagnosed or suspected, early intervention of expert help, such as orthopaedic or plastic surgeons (depending on the injury), is essential.

CONCLUSION

Extremity injuries are common following major trauma. The injuries may be life threatening requiring prompt assessment, resuscitation and expert help. Many extremity injuries have the potential to be limb threatening therefore careful assessment and examination is necessary. Subtle signs and symptoms mean that careful observation of the affected limb is essential. Other injuries, such as an intra-abdominal bleed or a subdural haematoma, may take priority over extremity trauma. Nevertheless, simple interventions in the ED such as early splinting, fracture realignment and wound irrigation will help to prevent long term disability for the patient.

KEY INFORMATION BOX

- Extremity injuries can look disturbing and be distracting – don't forget the assessment priorities!
- Bony injuries should be relocated or splinted as early as possible
- A wound over a swelling is an open fracture until proven otherwise – minimise infection risks
- The solution to pollution is dilution! Irrigate wounds early
- Check for haematuria in crush injured patients
- Pain, pallor, paraesthesia and paralysis? Think vascular or nerve injury or compartment syndrome
- Don't forget tetanus immunisation status.

REFERENCES

1. Greaves I, Porter KM, Ryan JM (Eds) (2001) Musculoskeletal trauma. In: Trauma care manual, 115–123. Arnold, London

2. American College of Surgeons Committee on Trauma (2004) Musculoskeletal trauma. Advanced trauma life support for doctors. Student course manual (7th edn), 205–219. American College of Surgeons, Chicago

3. Ziran BH, Freudigman (2002) Orthopaedic injuries. In: The trauma manual (2nd edn) (Eds Peitzman AB, Rhodes M, Schwab CW, Yealy DM, Fabian TC), 296–309. Lippincott, Williams & Wilkins, Philadelphia

4. Smith M (2005) Orthopaedic trauma. In: Principles and practice of trauma nursing (Ed O'Shea R), 379–419. Elsevier, Edinburgh

5. Davies KA (2002) Soft tissue trauma. In: The trauma manual (2nd edn) (Eds Peitzman AB, Rhodes M, Schwab CW, Yealy DM, Fabian TC), 352–355. Lippincott, Williams & Wilkins, Philadelphia

6. Hodgetts T, Turner L (2006) Trauma rules 2 (2nd edn), 121. Blackwell Publishing, Oxford

7. Department of Health (2006) Immunisation against infectious disease – 'The Green Book': Tetanus, chapter 30. http://www.dh.gov.uk/en/Policyandguidance/Healthand socialcaretopics/Greenbook/DH_4097254

8. Miller PR, Kane JM (2002) Compartment syndrome and rhabdomyolysis. In: The trauma manual (2nd edn) (Eds Peitzman AB, Rhodes M, Schwab CW, Yealy DM, Fabian TC), 335–339. Lippincott, Williams & Wilkins, Philadelphia

9. Demetriades D, Berne TV (2004) Extremity compartment syndrome. In: Assessment and management of trauma (Eds Demetriades D, Berne TV), 72–75. LAC & USC Healthcare Network, Los Angeles

10. Alarcon LH, Townsend RN (2002) Peripheral vascular injuries. In: The trauma manual (2nd edn) (Eds Peitzman AB, Rhodes M, Schwab CW, Yealy DM,

Fabian TC), 340–351. Lippincott, Williams & Wilkins, Philadelphia

11. Demetriades D, Berne TV (2004) Peripheral vascular injuries. In: Assessment and management of trauma (Eds Demetriades D, Berne TV), 54–55. LAC & USC Healthcare Network, Los Angeles

12. Bernard SL, Llull R, Nystrom NA (2002) Hand trauma. In: The trauma manual (2nd edn) (Eds Peitzman AB, Rhodes M, Schwab CW, Yealy DM, Fabian TC), 319–334. Lippincott, Williams & Wilkins, Philadelphia

Burns

9

Elaine Cole

Major burns are potentially life-threatening injuries.[1] Each year in the United Kingdom about 250,000 people sustain a burn. 3000 people require admission to hospital and in an average year 300 burn related deaths occur.[2]

Some burn victims will have an isolated burn (sometimes described as a thermal injury). However, associated traumatic injuries may be sustained during the burning event. For example, a burn victim may attempt to escape the fire by jumping from a burning building.[3] Similarly, a road traffic accident (RTA) where the vehicle caught fire or was involved in an explosion may also result in concurrent injuries. Therefore, regardless of mechanism of injury, as with any trauma patient, the initial assessment and resuscitation principles remain the same.

The aim of this chapter is to understand the principles of rapid assessment, resuscitation and stabilisation for the burn injured patient.

LEARNING OBJECTIVES
By the end of this chapter the reader will be able to:

- ❏ Identify the mechanism of burn injury
- ❏ Define the priorities for the victim of chemical or electrical burns
- ❏ Describe assessment and management priorities in relation to ABCDE
- ❏ Understand how to recognise burn depth, calculate burn surface area and calculate burn fluid formulae

❏ Identify which burn victims should be referred for specialist advice or treatment
❏ Describe priorities for transfer of the burn victim.

MECHANISM OF BURN INJURY

Burns have a number of causes, however by far the most common is heat, causing a thermal injury. The extent of the injury is dependent on the heat and the duration of the burn.[1]

Thermal burns can be further broken down into:

• Scalds (wet heat)
• Flame
• Contact (with hot surfaces).

Other causes of burns include:

• Chemical agents (alkali, acid or petroleum) causing a heat response
• Electricity producing heat and causing tissue and potential organ damage.

Chemical burns

Chemical burns can be caused by exposure to alkalis, acids or petroleum.[3,4] Alkali burns are considered to be more harmful than acids as they have the potential to penetrate skin and tissue more deeply.[3] The priority is to remove the chemical in order to stop the continued burning, damage and possible absorption of the chemical. This usually involves irrigation, sometimes for a prolonged period,[4] especially with alkalis. Skin can be tested with pH sticks following the period of irrigation to check that the pH is returning to neutral.

To minimise the risk of exposure to the chemical, ED staff involved in the care of the chemical burn victim should wear appropriate protective clothing. Specialist advice about the chemical and possible antidotes can be obtained online from the National Poisons Information Service via www.toxbase.co.uk

Electrical burns

Case study 9.1 Electrical burn injury

A 52-year-old man is brought to the ED. He had been trying to fix a broken computer at home and took the back off the computer casing without unplugging it from the mains. On touching the inside of the computer he sustained an electric shock, which caused him to fall from his chair to the floor.

On arrival at the ED he has a small white burn on his right hand covering most of his index finger. He is anxious and states that the injury is painless but that his hand and arm feel 'weird'. Other than this, he appears to be fine. Due to the nature of his injury the patient is referred to the plastic surgery registrar on call for review of what appears to be a full thickness finger burn.

After an hour in the department the patient starts to complain of chest pain and a fluttering feeling in his chest. A 12 lead ECG and the cardiac monitor both show a narrow complex tachycardia for which the patient requires admission.

Electrical burn injury can be difficult to detect. The source of the electrical power makes contact with the victim, and the resulting injury often depends on the voltage of the electrical current:[3]

- Low voltage (<1000 volts) from domestic mains supply (240 volts) and commercial industrial supply (415 volts). At these currents skin, subcutaneous tissue and deeper structures can be affected.
- High voltage (>1000 volts) can cause massive, devastating damage, both locally where the current enters the body and more widespread as the current travels through the body.

Looking at the outside of the body there may appear to be little damage, other than an entry burn and possibly an exit burn. However, as the electric current passes through the body, it causes heat and can burn skin, tissue, blood vessels, nerves and muscle. Complex problems can be caused, depending on the structures involved.

Cardiac involvement

If the electrical current has affected the heart, cardiac arrhythmias (abnormal heart rhythms) and myocardial ischaemia may occur. All electrical burn victims should have continuous cardiac monitoring and have a 12 lead ECG recorded to detect such problems.

Renal involvement

If muscle is burned or severely damaged, muscle protein (myoglobin) is released into the systemic circulation. Myoglobin is then filtered in the kidneys, causing damage to the glomerular filtration system, which may cause acute renal failure. Rhabdomyolysis, dark urine containing blood, is an indicator that this problem is occurring. Therefore urinalysis should be performed on all electrical burn victims. Intravenous fluids may need to be increased to ensure adequate renal function,[5] aiming for a urine output of 1–2 ml/kg/hour.

The burn victim with associated injuries

Burn victims can sustain associated injuries, depending on the mechanism and location of the incident:

- Jumping from a burning building can cause major orthopaedic, spinal cord and solid organ injuries.
- An RTA can cause multiple injuries, which may be compounded by burns if the vehicle ignited on impact.
- Blast injuries can be exacerbated by the presence of burns caused by ignition of the blast agent or the environment catching fire.
- Electrical injuries can cause falls and there can be violent tetanic muscle spasms resulting in fractures and soft tissue injury.[1]

Table 9.1 Important indicators in a history of burn injury

History	Relevance
Mechanism of injury	Risk of concurrent injuries
Burning agent	Potential burn depth Risk of other injuries (falls, chemical inhalation, etc.)
First aid measures	Cooling burn – limiting injury Irrigating chemicals
Time of burn	Intravenous fluid formulae are calculated using time of burn
Time in enclosed environment	Risk of inhalation injury Risk of carbon monoxide poisoning
Conscious level since injury	May indicate hypoxia, carbon monoxide poisoning, hypovolaemia
Inconsistent history of events	Non-accidental injury in children, the older person and vulnerable people Consider criminal intent
Past medical history	Exacerbating co-existing illnesses such as respiratory disease, heart failure, diabetes or suicidal intent

The nature of burn injuries and how they look means that they can be very distracting. It is essential that this potential distraction does not prevent other injuries being detected. Therefore, establishing a clear mechanism of injury and history of events is paramount.[4] Table 9.1 shows a summary of important indicators in the history. A systematic ABCDE assessment should be used to ensure that other injuries are not missed.

PRIMARY SURVEY ASSESSMENT AND RESUSCITATION

Airway with cervical spine control

The upper airway is susceptible to burns and the effects of inhaling hot gases from flame, smoke or steam.[1] The mucosa in the mouth and upper airway can swell very quickly following burn injury causing an airway obstruction.[6] When assessing the airway there should be a suspicion of airway obstruction and the airway should be reassessed frequently.

In the awake patient without airway compromise high flow oxygen, 15 L/min via a non-rebreathe mask, should be administered as a priority.

Signs of airway obstruction may not be obvious immediately[3] and therefore the presence of any of the following should alert the practitioner to possible airway compromise:

- Facial/neck burns
- Singed facial hair – beard, moustache, eyebrows, nasal hairs
- Burns to tongue/oropharynx
- Soot in the saliva or sputum
- Hoarseness/altered voice
- Stridor/noisy breathing
- Coughing
- History of confinement in heat
- Altered mental status – confusion or agitation.

If any of these are present then senior anaesthetic help should be urgently sought. The patient may need to have a definitive airway secured, with endotracheal intubation, before the swelling becomes too severe.[6]

Cervical spine immobilisation should be carried out if the mechanism of injury suggests that a potential cervical spine injury may have occurred.

Breathing and ventilation

Inhalation of hot gases, chemicals or products of combustion can compromise breathing and ventilation. Problems may be obvious or subtle but all have the potential to cause hypoxia, therefore early high flow oxygen is essential.

Dependent on the mechanism of injury and the type of burn that the patient has been exposed to, potential breathing problems caused by inhalation injury include:

- Bronchospasm (causing a wheeze or noisy breathing)
- Pulmonary oedema (causing difficulty in breathing, poor saturations and increasing hypoxia)

- Carbon monoxide poisoning (causing an altered mentation, from anxiety, confusion through to unconsciousness)
- Pneumonia (a later problem but signs of hypoxia should be observed for).

If any of these problems are suspected, senior medical help should be sought immediately. In order to detect potential or actual problems with breathing and ventilation, assessment should include:

- Respiratory rate
- Chest movement and depth
- Listening for the presences of a wheeze or stridor
- Noting burns to the chest (front and back) that may impede chest movement
- Altered mentation – anxiety or confusion
- Oxygen saturation monitoring (although with caution as the machine cannot tell the difference between haemoglobin with oxygen and haemoglobin with carbon monoxide)
- Arterial blood gas measurement.

To maximise oxygenation and control breathing problems the patient may be sedated, intubated and ventilated at an early stage. This decision will be made by a senior clinician based on the patient's physiological status and the arterial blood gas results.

Carbon monoxide poisoning

Carbon monoxide (CO) is an odourless, colourless gas.[4] Once inhaled it has a much stronger affinity for combining with haemoglobin than oxygen (240 times greater).[3] When carbon monoxide binds with haemoglobin it forms carboxyhaemaglobin (COHb). The COHb reduces the capacity for blood to carry oxygen, in fact it displaces the oxygen from the haemoglobin and this results in tissue hypoxia.[4]

Burn victims who have been confined in an enclosed space are at risk of CO poisoning. Signs and symptoms of CO poisoning may be very subtle, therefore anyone who has been confined during a burn injury is at risk and should be investigated and treated as such.

The principle treatment of CO poisoning is high flow oxygen. Blood should be taken for carboxyhaemaglobin levels but oxygen should not be delayed whilst the results are waited for.

Symptoms of CO poisoning are generally linked to the COHb levels in the blood stream:[1,3,4]

- COHb 15–30% – tiredness, anxiety, irritability, nausea, headache
- COHb 30–40% – confusion, vomiting, dizziness
- COHb 40–60% – signs of shock, tachycardia, tachypnoea, convulsions, coma
- COHb >60% – coma, cardiorespiratory arrest.

Treatment of CO poisoning

As previously mentioned, first line treatment is early high flow oxygen, 15 L/min via a non-rebreathe mask.

Carbon monoxide dissociates very slowly and has a half-life of 250 minutes or 4 hours whilst the patient is breathing room air (21%).[3] If high flow oxygen is administered then the half-life reduces to 40 minutes.

In severe cases of CO poisoning the patient may be treated in a hyperbaric oxygen chamber. Here, oxygen is forced back onto the haemoglobin displacing the CO. Hyperbaric oxygenation may be considered for the following:[6]

- Unconsciousness at scene
- COHb levels of >30%
- Pregnancy.

Circulation and haemorrhage control

Circulation should be assessed as for any trauma patient. The following vital signs should be monitored to detect circulatory problem:

- Heart rate
- Blood pressure

- Capillary refill time
- Level of consciousness
- Cardiac monitoring is indicated for the electrical burn victim.

Fluid loss and fluid replacement in burns

Patients with partial and full thickness burns loose fluid because of increased cellular and vascular permeability.[4] The normal inflammatory response as a result of the burn injury means that mediators, such as histamine, cause the cells and vessels to become 'leaky' with fluid moving from inside the cells to outside of the cells. Visible fluid loss can also be seen in exudate and blistering.[4]

The fluid loss described above occurs over the first 8–12 hours following the burn injury.[4,7] Therefore if the patient initially appears to be in hypovolaemic shock this may be due to an associated injury and should not be attributed to the burn in the early stages of the assessment.

When deciding if the burn injured patient needs intravenous fluids the following needs to be considered:

- Burn depth
- Burn surface area
- The age of the patient
- Fluid replacement formulae.

Burn depth

The skin is made up of a number of layers (Figure 9.1). The extent to which the skin layers are involved will determine burn depth (Table 9.2). Burns are rarely uniform and a mixed pattern of burn depth will be seen.[1] In Figure 9.2 partial thickness burns (near to the edge of the burn, darker in colour) can be seen around a large full thickness burn (lighter in colour).

- Superficial burns, where the skin is reddened but intact, somewhat like sunburn, intravenous fluids are not indicated

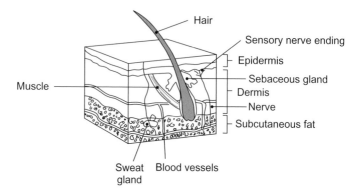

Fig. 9.1 Cross section of the skin

Table 9.2 Burn depth

Depth of burn	Clinical signs
Superficial: epidermal involvement	Painful, pink or red skin
Partial thickness: involving the epidermis and dermis	Red skin, thin walled blisters, moist broken skin, very painful, blisters may form over a number of hours
Deep dermal: burn involves the epidermis, dermis and deep dermis	Painful, blistering, may look paler than partial thickness, may be dry
Full thickness: burn involves all layers of the skin and may include subcutaneous fat, muscle, blood vessels and bone	Painless, hard, no blisters, white/grey/blackened appearance

- Partial thickness burns are deeper, where the skin is broken and blistered and fluid can be lost
- Full thickness burns where the skin, fat, muscle, blood vessels and even bone can be involved require surgery and skin grafting.[4]

Both partial thickness and full thickness burns may require intravenous fluids depending on the burn surface area.

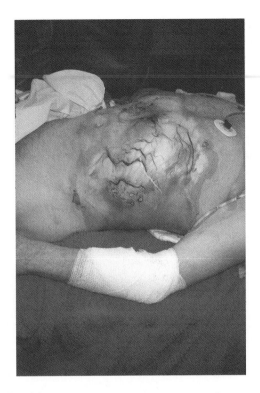

Fig. 9.2 Burn injury

Burn surface area

Burn surface area (BSA) means the total area of the body that has been burnt. Burns are rarely sustained in a neat easily measurable pattern and it can be a challenge to work out how much of the surface of the body is involved. Three methods for deciding BSA are:[1,4]

- The Rule of Nines
- The Lund and Browder Chart
- The patient's palm measurement.

The Rule of Nines broadly divides the body up into multiples of 9. The Lund and Browder chart[8] (Figure 9.3) divides the body into numerical sections and allows for percentage of partial and full thickness involvement to be documented. The patient's palmar surface area represents 1% of the patient's body surface area.[3] Using this as a rough guide, a paper

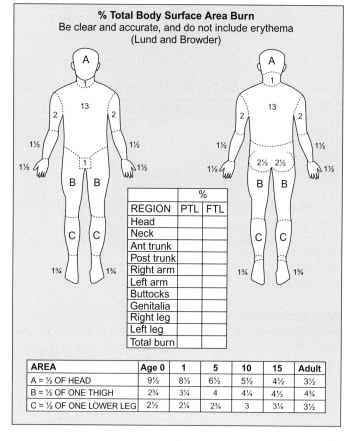

% Total Body Surface Area Burn
Be clear and accurate, and do not include erythema
(Lund and Browder)

REGION	% PTL	FTL
Head		
Neck		
Ant trunk		
Post trunk		
Right arm		
Left arm		
Buttocks		
Genitalia		
Right leg		
Left leg		
Total burn		

AREA	Age 0	1	5	10	15	Adult
A = ½ OF HEAD	9½	8½	6½	5½	4½	3½
B = ½ OF ONE THIGH	2¾	3¼	4	4¼	4½	4¾
C = ½ OF ONE LOWER LEG	2½	2¼	2¾	3	3¼	3½

Fig. 9.3 The Lund and Browder chart[8]

template could be cut to size and this may be a useful way of estimating BSA where the burns are irregularly spread across the body.

The age of the burn injured patient

The age of the patient together with the burn depth and BSA will determine if the patient needs intravenous fluid replacement.[9]

Superficial reddening of the skin, or eythema, is not included in the BSA for fluid replacement.

- Children with >10% partial or full thickness burns will need intravenous fluids.
- Adults with >15% partial or full thickness burns will need intravenous fluids.

Fluid replacement formulae

The burn injured patient should have two large bore cannulae inserted. It is possible to cannulate through burned skin but this should be avoided if possible.[1,7] Blood tests as for any trauma patient should be requested (see Chapter 2). These should also include carboxyhaemaglobin levels and a haematocrit (to determine plasma loss).

Several fluid formulae for burns exist, however in Britain the Parkland formula is most commonly advocated:[1,4]

- $4 \times BSA \times$ weight in kg = ml of crystalloid to be infused over the first 24 hours
- Half of the fluid should be given over 8 hours from the time of the burn
- Half of the fluid should be given over the remaining 16 hours, adjusted as per the patient's physiological status and urine output

Crystalloid solutions such as Hartmanns or 0.9% Saline are administered in the first 24 hours post burn injury[2] to ensure cardiovascular stability and normal urine output. The fluids may be changed to colloids after the first 24 hours due to oedema formation.[10]

Case study 9.2 Intravenous fluids for burn injury

An 18-year-old woman has sustained 35% partial and full thickness burns as a result of a fire in a nightclub. She needs intravenous fluid replacement and the Parkland formula will be used. Her weight is estimated at 60 kg.
Her fluid requirements are calculated thus:

$$4 \times 35 \text{ (BSA)} \times 60 \text{ (weight in kg)} = 8400 \text{ ml of Hartmanns solution}$$

The burn injury occurred at 01.00 and it is now 02.00 in the ED. As the injury occurred an hour ago the first half of the fluid (4200 ml) needs to be given over 7 hours to fit within the first 8 hour period.

Children under 30 kg in weight require maintenance fluids in addition to the burn injury fluids.[7] This is because they have a higher blood volume per kilo than adults. Glucose is used for the maintenance fluids as children have lower stores of glycogen and are more at risk of hypoglycaemia.[4]

Urine output should be carefully monitored in all patients receiving intravenous fluids. This will help to monitor the efficacy of the fluid replacement to avoid over- or underresuscitation.[1] A urinary catheter should be inserted and the following minimum urine output aimed for:

- Adults – 0.5 ml/kg/hour
- Children – 1 ml/kg/hour
- Infants – 2 ml/kg/hour.

If urine output is less than these volumes it may indicate that more fluids are needed. Senior medical advice should be sought urgently.

In larger burns >25% BSA it is optimal to obtain central venous access early. This should be performed by a senior clinician under strict asepsis. A central venous catheter (CVC) allows for rapid fluid replacement. Additionally it assists in monitoring the central fluid balance through measurement of the central venous pressure (CVP).[11]

Disability and dysfunction
An altered level of consciousness may indicate one or more of the following:

- Hypoxia
- Inhalation injury
- Carbon monoxide poisoning
- Hypovolaemia
- An associated head injury
- Hypoglycaemia
- Alcohol or drug ingestion.

The level of consciousness should be assessed regularly and any reduction or alteration reported to a senior clinician. A blood sugar measurement should be taken and if an associated head injury is suspected, regular monitoring of the Glasgow Coma Scale (GCS) and pupilliary response.

Exposure and environmental control
The patient should be fully undressed with all clothing, jewellery and other restricting items removed. This may have already been done on the patient's arrival, to help with irrigation and cooling. A number of areas need to be considered in 'exposure and environmental control':

- Analgesia (if pain has not yet been assessed and analgesia administered)
- Tetanus immunity
- Temperature control
- Wound care
- A nasogastric tube.

Analgesia for the burn injured patient
Burns can cause severe pain and a great deal of fear and anxiety for the patient. Analgesia should be considered in the

early stages of assessment and its effects monitored regularly. It is suggested that full thickness burns are painless, as nerves have been damaged, however at the edges of all full thickness burns there are extremely painful partial thickness and superficial burns[4] (Figure 9.2).

Intravenous opiate analgesia such as morphine should be given, with doses titrated to the patient's pain. An antiemetic should also be given at the same time. The intravenous route works quickly and effectively.

Tetanus immunisation

As the skin has been breached the patient is at risk of tetanus infection. The patient, if conscious, should be asked about their tetanus immunity. If they do not have adequate coverage, a tetanus toxoid booster should be administered.[12] If there is doubt about the immunity of an unconscious patient then a booster can be administered.

Temperature control

The risk of hypothermia in the burn injured patient is often overlooked.[1] Copious irrigation and cooling with wet soaks can cause hypothermia. Heat loss can be significant through the broken skin,[7] therefore it is preferable to cover the patient's unaffected areas as soon as possible to minimise systemic cooling. Once the burns have been assessed they should be covered as described below.

Wound care

Burns should be cooled and irrigated as per injury type. In the ED the preferred method of covering a burn prior to surgery or transfer is either with a film such as cling film or a film dressing such as Tegaderm™ or Opsite™. Alternatively a clean dry sheet may be a suitable alternative.

Full thickness burns, even if small in BSA, need to be referred for specialist assessment as they may require surgical debridement and skin grafting. Other burned areas of the body that may cause concern and require specialist referral include:[4,9]

- The ears – poor blood supply with potentially delayed healing
- The eyes – risk of loss of vision and eyelid function
- The genitals, perineum and rectum – risk of infection and delayed healing
- Joint surfaces – risk of contractures and mobility problems.

Nasogastric tube placement

In severe burns of more than 20–25% BSA there is a risk of developing a paralytic ileus, which is a disruption of normal gastrointestinal activity.[13] The patient may feel nauseated, vomit or experience abdominal pain/distension, therefore gastric decompression is necessary. A nasogastric tube should be passed[1,3,7] and the stomach contents aspirated to avoid the risk of vomiting and aspiration into the lungs.

REFERRAL AND TRANSFER

A burn injured patient may have associated traumatic injuries that are more life threatening than the burn injury, such as an extradural haematoma or an unstable pelvic fracture. These will need to be dealt with before transferring the patient, however specialist advice from a burns and plastics unit should be sought.

Once other injuries have been assessed and managed or excluded, the burn injury may need referral or transfer for specialist help.

Referral

The local burns unit should be contacted for advice and guidance about burn injury management, especially for potentially complex issues including.[9]

- Partial or full thickness burns >10% BSA in an adult
- Partial or full thickness burns >5% BSA in a child
- Burns involving potentially problematic areas: neck, face, axilla, hands, feet, joints, eyes, ears, genitalia, perineum, rectum

- Chemical burns
- Electrical burns
- Inhalation injury
- Circumferential burns (burns that encircle a whole digit, limb or torso area where there is a risk to function)
- Burns in patients at the extreme of ages (<5 years or >60 years)
- Burns in patients with significant pre-existing medical conditions, e.g. cardiovascular disease, respiratory disease or diabetes.

Transfer

Transferring any patient from one hospital to another carries a risk, however as most burns units are located some distance from a general ED the transfer of a burns patient needs careful planning and preparation. The escorting practitioner will vary depending on resources available and local policy. Ideally it should be an experienced nurse or doctor who is able to assess the patient and intervene if necessary during the transfer.

Table 9.3 shows the areas that need to be considered prior to transfer.

CONCLUSION

Burns can be caused by a number of agents, some of which, such as chemical or electrical burns, will result in the patient having complex assessment and management needs. The burn victim may have sustained other injuries, therefore systematic ABCDE assessment is needed to ensure that nothing is missed. Priorities during the initial assessment and management of the burn injured patient include airway assessment and stabilisation, high flow oxygen delivery, burn cooling and irrigation and effective analgesia. The need for intravenous fluid resuscitation depends on burn depth and burn surface area. Early advice from a specialist burns unit is recommended to ensure the correct definitive care and treatment for the burn injured patient.

Table 9.3 Transfer considerations for the burn injured patient

Consideration	Details
Referral	Person to person referral is essential. The doctor in charge of the burn victim's care must speak in person to the accepting doctor at the burns unit. The plan of care on route, any specific instructions and the name of the receiving doctor and ward must be documented in the patient's notes
Airway	The patient's airway must be assessed by a senior clinician prior to transfer. The patient may need to be intubated if there is any risk of potential airway compromise
Analgesia	Prior to moving the patient the need for more analgesia should be assessed. The escorting nurse or doctor should take extra analgesia for administration during the transfer journey if necessary
Lines and tubes	All should be checked prior to moving the patient. This should include: Oxygen mask and supply Intravenous cannulae are securely fastened and fluids available Urinary catheter and hourly drainage bag NG tube and drainage bag
Equipment	This may be provided by the pre-hospital care team, however the escorting practitioner should ensure that the following is available: Suction equipment Airway adjuncts and a bag valve mask device Cardiac monitoring Resuscitation drugs
Documentation	All of the patient assessment and management should be clearly documented including: Vital signs Fluid balance chart Burns chart Past medical history and allergies (if known) Next of kin and contact details Property and valuables

KEY INFORMATION BOX

- Stop the burning process, cool and/or irrigate the burn early (beware of causing hypothermia!)
- All burn injured patients need high flow oxygen
- Burns do not cause hypotension and tachycardia in the early stages following the injury – is the patient bleeding somewhere?
- The airway needs to be assessed and reassessed regularly – have a high index of suspicion of airway compromise
- An altered level of consciousness should cause suspicion of COHb poisoning
- Calculate burn depth and BSA to determine if the patient needs intravenous fluids
- Monitor urine output to assess fluid resuscitation
- Transfer of a burn injured patient is a high risk procedure and needs careful planning and preparation.

REFERENCES

1. Greaves I, Porter KM, Ryan JM (Eds) (2001) Injuries due to burns and cold. In: Trauma care manual, 205–218. Arnold, London

2. Hettiaratchy S, Dziewulski P (2004) Clinical review. ABC of burns. BMJ 328:1366–1368

3. American College of Surgeons (2004) Injuries due to burns and cold. In: Advanced trauma life support for doctors. Student course manual (7th edn), 231–242. American College of Surgeons, Chicago

4. Jenkins L (2005) Care of the patient with major burns. In: Principles and practice of trauma nursing (Ed O'Shea R), 497–512. Elsevier, Edinburgh

5. Miller PR, Kane JM (2002) Compartment syndrome and rhabdomyolysis. In: The trauma manual (2nd edn) (Eds Peitzman AB, Rhodes M, Schwab CW, Yealy DM, Fabian TC), 335–339. Lippincott, Williams & Wilkins, Philadelphia

6. Hodgetts T, Turner L (2006) Trauma rules 2 (2nd edn), 44–45. Blackwell Publishing, Oxford

7. Farrell K, Haith LR (2002) Burns/inhalation. In: The trauma manual (2nd edn) (Eds Peitzman AB, Rhodes M, Schwab CW, Yealy DM, Fabian TC), 433–445. Lippincott, Williams & Wilkins, Philadelphia

8. Lund C, Browder N (1944) The estimation of areas of burns. Surgery, Gynecology and Obstetrics 79:352–358

9. British Burn Association (2003) National referral guidelines. http://www.britishburnassociation.co.uk/

10. Cancio LC, Chavez S, Alvarado-Ortega M, Barillo DJ, Walker S, McManus AT, Goodwin CW (2004) Predicting increased fluid requirements during the resuscitation of thermally injured patients. Journal of Trauma, Injury, Infection and Critical Care 56:404–414

11. Cole E (2007) Measuring central venous pressure. Nursing Standard 22(7):40–42

12. Department of Health (2006) Immunisation against infectious disease – 'The Green Book': tetanus, chapter 30. http://www.dh.gov.uk/en/Policyandguidance/Healthand socialcaretopics/Greenbook/DH_4097254

13. Rose D, Jordan EB (1999) Perioperative management of burn patients. AORN Journal 69:1208–1230

10 Paediatric Trauma

Joanna Hall

INTRODUCTION

Paediatric trauma is responsible for the greatest number of deaths in the paediatric population and as such it is vital that the emergency department practitioner is competent in their management. In 2005 two million children were admitted to emergency departments (ED) in England and Wales as a result of trauma, resulting in 251 deaths in patients under the age of 15. There has however been a steady decrease in the number of paediatric trauma deaths over the last two decades, illustrated by the data for 1979 when 1100 children died.[1] This steady decrease in the number of paediatric trauma deaths can be partly attributable to the improvements and advances in resuscitation and management but it is also due to the recognition and increased profile of accident prevention strategies resulting in fewer incidents of paediatric unintentional injury.

The aim of this chapter is to understand the principles of the rapid assessment, resuscitation and stabilisation of seriously injured children.

LEARNING OBJECTIVES

By the end of this chapter the reader will be able to:

❑ Identify differences in normal physiological parameters for children according to age
❑ Identify the major differences in injury patterns in paediatric trauma patients

❏ Adapt the ABCDE assessment approach for paediatric trauma patients
❏ Identify psychosocial issues affecting the paediatric trauma patient and manage them accordingly.

MECHANISMS OF INJURY

Blunt trauma is more prevalent than penetrating trauma in children. Falls are the most common mechanism of injury and reason for attendance at the ED but result in few deaths. Road traffic accidents (RTA) account for the most deaths and serious injuries, with drowning and burns being the next most prevalent causes of injury. The incidence of penetrating trauma usually associated with knives and firearms increases in the teenage population.

The priorities of assessment and management of the injured child are the same as in the adult, however their unique anatomical, physiological and psychological characteristics in combination with their particular mechanism of injury produce distinct patterns of injury. For example, during an RTA, a car bumper would potentially impact with the head of a small child and cause a different pattern of injuries than the same incident involving an adult. In addition, the ranges of normal physiological parameters such as cardiovascular observations change with age and it is imperative that the ED practitioner is able to accurately measure and interpret these parameters. Normal physiological observations can be found in Table 10.1.

Table 10.1 Normal paediatric observation parameters according to age

Age (years)	RR (breaths per minute)	HR (beats per minute)	Systolic BP (mmHg)
<1	30–40	110–160	70–90
1–2	25–35	100–150	80–95
2–5	25–30	95–140	80–100
5–12	20–25	80–120	90–110
>12	15–20	60–100	100–120

> **Box 10.1 Weight estimation based on age**
>
> Weight (kg) = (Age (years) + 4) × 2

The smaller size of the child, the relative reduction in body fat, proximity of multiple organs and increase in elasticity of their tissues results in greater force applied per unit of body area and the transfer of that energy to different body parts. As a result multiple organ injuries are common and the proportionately large head in younger children results in a higher incidence of blunt brain injuries in this age group.

The body surface area to body volume ratio is highest at birth and decreases with age, resulting in the potentially rapid development of hypothermia which may further complicate the management of the traumatised child. The weight of the child increases with age and it is often necessary to estimate it, as obtaining an accurate weight is often impractical. If the age of the child is unknown, use of a Broselow tape laid alongside the child uses the child's length to estimate weight and is relatively accurate. The formula in Box 10.1 is a useful tool in weight estimations where the age of the child is known and can be used for children aged between 1 and 10 years. It also has the advantage of allowing an estimated weight to be calculated before the child's arrival in hospital, which will allow time to estimate fluids and drug requirements.[2–4]

ANATOMICAL AND PHYSIOLOGICAL DIFFERENCES IN CHILDREN

Airway
Apart from the obvious smaller size of the airway, the paediatric patient has a number of anatomical and physiological differences that will ultimately affect their management.

- Children aged <3 years have to breathe through their nose: secretions or blood in the nasal passages will impede breathing.
- Large occiput and short flexible trachea: partial obstruction of the airway results when the child is supine.
- Funnel shaped trachea: secretions and foreign bodies more easily accumulated in the back of the mouth, loose teeth, blood and secretions can have serious consequences.
- Cricoid ring is narrowest part of the airway not the larynx: area is susceptible to oedema, uncuffed endotracheal tubes are preferred to minimise pressure on mucosal lining at the cricoid ring although there is some evidence which challenges this practice.[5]
- Large tongue and tonsils in comparison to the oral cavity, epiglottis and larynx have a different shape and position: intubation may be easier using a straight bladed laryngoscope.
- Shorter length of trachea: the endotracheal tube may be placed in the right main bronchus or dislodged, it is therefore essential to monitor the intubated child for bilateral chest movement.[3]

Cervical spine

As in the adult, unless the mechanism of injury clearly excludes the possibility of a cervical spine injury, spinal precautions must be implemented from the outset. Cervical spine injuries in children are associated with substantial levels of force but remain relatively rare accounting for less than 2% of all spinal fractures and dislocations in children.[4] Due to the comparatively large head of the small child flexion or forward bending of the C-spine occurs at a higher level than in the adult and as a result the upper three vertebrae of the cervical spine are usually involved in any injury.[6]

Breathing

The anatomical and physiological differences associated with breathing in the child are more than just a difference in size of the airways, although it is important to remember that additional decreases in the diameter of the airways will have significant effects. Hypoxia is the most common cause of cardiac arrest in children and it is vital that adequate ventilation is achieved at all times.

- Compliant chest wall with horizontally lying ribs: ribs contribute less to chest expansion, compliant chest wall allows significant damage to be done to underlying lung tissue even in the absence of rib fractures. Extreme force is required to cause multiple rib fractures and the associated underlying damage is usually very severe, flail segments are poorly tolerated for this reason.
- Fewer type 1 muscle fibres (slow-twitch, fatigue resistant); fatigue appears earlier in increased work of breathing. Recession is seen relatively easily in smaller children and is a good indicator of respiratory distress. A silent chest is a pre-terminal sign and indicates imminent cardiac arrest if not appropriately and rapidly managed.
- More mobile mediastinal structures which may result in earlier tracheal deviation in tension pneumothorax and massive haemothorax.
- Increased metabolic rate results in an increased oxygen demand and as such normal respiratory rates are higher in children, decreasing with age. Oxygen saturation monitoring is useful to determine the efficacy of ventilation but beware of its accuracy when used on cold digits, highly mobile children or in severe hypoxia, as monitors become less accurate when oxygen saturations fall below 80%.[7]

Circulation

The child has a larger circulating volume per kilogram than the adult (70–80 ml/kg) but their total circulating volume remains relatively small, meaning a minor amount of blood loss can be significant. The infant has a fixed stroke volume so cardiac output may only be increased by increasing the heart rate. The normal parameters of heart rates in children

---

Box 10.2 Estimated systolic blood pressure

Systolic BP = 80 + (2 × age)

---

decrease with age whilst stroke volume increases as a result of the growing heart.[8]

The primary response to hypovolaemia in the child is tachycardia. Changes to tissue perfusion, pulse pressure, level of consciousness and skin temperature occur later. Blood pressure is well maintained in the hypovolaemic child, however a narrowing pulse pressure, which is the difference between the systolic and diastolic blood pressure, to less than 20 mmHg is significant. The lower limit of normal systolic blood pressure in a child can be calculated using the formula in Box 10.2.

Hypotension is a pre-terminal sign and indicates a loss of more than 45% of the total circulating volume.[4] It is often accompanied by bradycardia and indicates imminent cardiac arrest.

Sites of bleeding in children generally remain the same as in the adult with one exception. In the child under 1 year of age, scalp wounds may bleed sufficiently enough to cause hypovolaemia.

Abdominal injuries are common, particularly those involving the liver and spleen. The horizontally lying rib cage, flatter diaphragm and thin abdominal wall means that these organs lie lower and are given less protection by the ribs and are therefore more susceptible to injury. In addition the bladder sits in the abdomen rather than the pelvis making it more vulnerable to damage when full.[7]

Disability
Head injury is a common cause of death in the paediatric population accounting for 25% of deaths in the 5 to 15 year age group.[4]

- Cranial suture lines remain unfused until approximately 18 months increasing the capacity of the cranial cavity. Children under this age may have significant injuries or bleeding without obvious neurological signs and symptoms and should be closely monitored for deterioration. After this age the cranial cavity behaves in the same way as that of the adult.
- Smaller subarachnoid space where CSF flows cushioning the brain, offers less protection to the underlying brain tissue. Cerebral blood flow is twice that of an adult by the time the child is 5 years but then starts to decrease. This increased blood flow partly explains the paediatric patient's severe susceptibility to cerebral hypoxia and highlights the need for the provision and maintenance of high flow oxygen to prevent secondary brain injury.[4]

PRIMARY SURVEY, ASSESSMENT AND RESUSCITATION

Airway

Initial assessment of the paediatric airway follows the same principles as in the adult, however specific paediatric considerations include:

- The head should be carefully positioned whilst maintaining manual cervical spine immobilisation to ensure that partial airway obstruction does not occur due to the child's large occiput.
- The airway should be inspected for the presence of secretions, blood or foreign bodies and removed using suction under direct supervision. Overzealous or deep suctioning may cause vagus nerve stimulation and result in bradycardia.
- Visible foreign bodies may be removed using small Magill's forceps but blind finger sweeps or use of instruments to remove invisible objects may serve to worsen the problem due to the child's funnel shaped trachea.

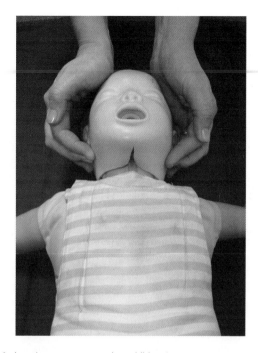

Fig. 10.1 Jaw thrust manoeuvre in a child

- Jaw thrust manoeuvre may also be used to support the child's airway but care should be taken to ensure pressure is placed only on the bony prominences and not on the soft tissues to avoid compressing the tongue and causing airway obstruction. Figure 10.1 illustrates the correct technique for performing a jaw thrust in a child.
- Oropharyngeal airways (Guedel) are useful in the unconscious child and are sized using the same method as in the adult. In children under the age of 5 the airway should be inserted with the concave side downwards using a tongue depressor in order to avoid causing any damage to the soft palate.

- Nasopharyngeal airways are often better tolerated in children but should only be used once an anterior base of skull fracture has been excluded. Sizing and insertion remains the same as in the adult.

Placement of a definitive airway should only be performed by a trained clinician, however it is the ED practitioner's role to assist with intubation. Due to the anatomical differences in the child it is often easier to use a straight bladed laryngoscope in small children which is designed to lift the epiglottis to enable visualisation of the vocal cords. The potential disadvantage of this method is that it may cause vagus nerve stimulation resulting in laryngospasm or bradycardia.

Uncuffed endotracheal tubes are preferred in children up until approximately 8–10 years of age in order to prevent damage to the tracheal mucosa. An appropriately sized tube should allow for a small air leak to avoid pressure from the tube on the mucosal lining and failure to observe this may result in damage to the cricoid ring and subsequent oedema following extubation. Sizing an endotracheal tube in a child may be performed using the formulae in Table 10.2 but are only suitable for use in the child over 1 year of age.[3] Children under this age usually require a tube of internal diameter 3.0–3.5 mm. In addition to the selected tube size, the clinician should also prepare one a size larger and one a size smaller in case the original tube proves to be too large or small.

Once successful intubation has occurred and correct placement of the endotracheal tube established, end tidal carbon dioxide monitoring should be commenced to ensure that ventilation is adequate.

In total airway obstruction such as facial burns or fractures where intubation cannot occur, needle cricothyroidotomy is

Table 10.2 Endotracheal tube length and diameter calculation

Internal diameter (mm)	(Age/4) + 4
Length (cm) oral tube	(Age/2) + 12
Length (cm) nasal tube	(Age/2) + 15

preferred and should be performed in all children under the age of 12. Surgical cricothyroidotomy is rarely indicated in this age group and it is difficult to palpate the cricothyroid membrane in children younger than this. Jet insufflation can be achieved using smaller quantities of oxygen than would usually be delivered to trauma patients to minimise the risk of barotrauma resulting from overinflation of the lungs. The child should receive 1 L/min of oxygen for each year of age and this should be delivered using the same technique as described in Chapter 2.

Cervical spine immobilisation

Case study 10.1 Cervical spine immobilisation in children

A 6-year-old child has been involved in a road traffic accident. On arrival to the ED he is irritable, crying and obviously distressed despite the presence of his mother. From this it is apparent that his airway is patent and the nurse applies 15 litres of oxygen via a non-rebreathe mask. He becomes more distressed when the nurse tries to lie him down and apply a cervical spine collar. This poses a real challenge: how should his cervical spine be immobilised?

Cervical spine injury should be assumed in all injured children and as a result the spine should be immobilised from the outset. The gold standard for children remains either:

- Manual immobilisation OR
- Collar, blocks and tape.

However, this can be extremely difficult in conscious children because they do not like being forcibly held down and often some flexibility is required. Traditional immobilisation techniques can be distressing for the child and struggling may cause increased movement in the neck increasing the risk of additional damage to any existing injury. If the conscious

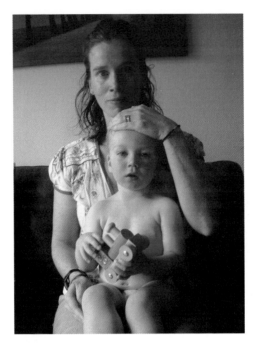

Fig. 10.2 Cervical spine immobilisation in the distressed child

child will tolerate a rigid collar only but lie still on a bed and not move then this is often the safer approach than either manually immobilising their neck or using additional equipment. In the extremely distressed child it may not even be possible to encourage the child to lie flat on the bed and these children are best managed by leaving them in a position where they will remain as still and calm as possible which is often sitting on a parent's or carer's lap (Figure 10.2). It is important that the child is treated in as calm and supportive atmosphere as possible and the use of distraction techniques or involvement of the hospital play specialist if available may assist in the management of the cervical spine.

Breathing

Hypoxia is the commonest cause of cardiorespiratory arrest in children and it is imperative that optimum ventilation is achieved from the outset. Assessment of breathing follows the same principles as in the adult, however the paediatric patient will display additional signs of respiratory distress:

- Accessory muscle use: sternomastoid, abdominal muscles
- Recession: subcostal, intercostal, sternal
- Nasal flaring
- Tracheal tug.

In the spontaneously breathing child 15 L/min oxygen should be administered using a paediatric non-rebreathe mask as soon as the airway is cleared. If ventilatory support is required then bag-valve-mask ventilation should be commenced with supplementary oxygen. An appropriately sized bag and well fitting mask should be used to reduce the risk of barotrauma and maximise ventilation. The various bag-valve-mask sizes can be found in Table 10.3.

Crying children or those who have been placed on a positive pressure ventilator will accumulate air in their stomachs. This splints and restricts the diaphragm and ultimately reduces the efficacy of respiration. The stomach should be decompressed by placement of an orogastric tube or nasogastric tube once basal skull fracture has been excluded.

Recognition of chest trauma remains the same in the children as for adults, although percussion may have limited value due to the general hyperresonance of the child's chest.

Table 10.3 Appropriate sizes for bag-valve-mask ventilation

Age	Size of bag
<1	250 ml
1–10	500 ml
>10	1000 ml

Absence of rib fractures does not exclude significant chest trauma due to the compliant chest wall and indeed the presence of rib fractures will suggest significant forces have been involved. Landmarks for intervention for needle decompression and chest drain insertion remain the same, although smaller equipment will be required.

Circulation and haemorrhage control

Assessment of circulation follows the same principles as described for the adult patient. The primary response to hypovolaemia will be tachycardia; other physiological signs do not appear until later. These include:

- Capillary refill time is a useful indicator of tissue perfusion in children and should be performed centrally on the sternum by applying digital pressure for 5 seconds and then releasing. The tissue should return to its normal colour within 2 seconds. Anything longer than this is considered delayed and if accompanied by tachycardia is indicative of hypovolaemia.[3]
- Blood pressure is well maintained during the early stages of hypovolaemia, however it is vital that accurate measurements are recorded to monitor for a narrowing pulse pressure. An appropriately sized cuff that covers 80% of the child's upper arm should be used.[3]

Intravenous access should be established with the placement of two relatively large bore cannulae if possible. The paediatric patient who is haemodynamically compromised due to haemorrhage can be difficult to cannulate and intraosseous needle insertion may be required if the situation is urgent or if other options have failed. Instructions and an illustration of the insertion of an intraosseous needle can be found in Box 10.3 and Figure 10.3.

There is some evidence that overzealous fluid administration in adult patients following trauma may be harmful in the presence of uncontrolled bleeding and whilst there is not the

---

Box 10.3 Intraosseous needle insertion

- May be used on all ages but increasingly difficult when bones start to calcify, realistically it is often only possible to insert them in children under 6 years old
- Preferred site for insertion is in the proximal tibia, approximately 2 cm below the tibial tuberosity on the medial aspect where a flattened section of bone can be felt close to the surface of the skin
- Successful insertion results in a 'give' as the needle penetrates the cortex and enters the marrow. Small volumes of marrow may be aspirated and analysed for most laboratory tests with the exception of blood gases
- Virtually all fluids and drugs can be infused; however they must always be 'pushed' as gravity will not provide sufficient force for infusion
- Contraindicated with proximal fractures and alternative sites may need to be used. Other sites for insertion are the distal, lateral aspect of the femur, iliac crest and sternum

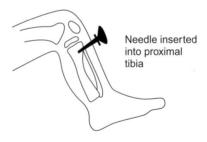

Needle inserted into proximal tibia

Fig. 10.3 Intraosseous needle insertion

same evidence for its use in children it is appropriate to follow similar cautious guidelines. Rapid restoration of blood pressure may disrupt early clot formation with subsequent increases in bleeding. Focusing on the administration of fluid rather than the cause of bleeding may delay much needed surgical intervention.

When a fluid bolus is indicated it should be given in *10 ml/ kg aliquots of 0.9% normal saline with careful reassessment after each aliquot*.

The need for emergency surgical intervention to control bleeding should also be considered at the outset and urgently sought if 20 ml/kg of fluid has not stabilised the child. *If 40 ml/kg of fluid has been administered to the child, half of their total circulating volume will have been replaced*. If haemodynamic instability remains, fluid replacement should be continued with blood in the volume of 10 ml/kg.

If a child is haemodynamically unstable the priority is to find the bleeding and seek expert surgical help.

Urinary catheterisation should be performed in the haemodynamically unstable child in order to monitor renal perfusion and to determine the adequacy of fluid resuscitation. Normal urine output in the child is significantly higher than in the adult:

- Infants <1 year: 2 ml/kg/hour
- Children >1 year: 1 ml/kg/hour.

Disability

The principles outlined in Chapter 3 are applicable to children but is important to identify some additional points:

- Children are more susceptible to secondary brain injury than adults due to their increased cerebral blood flow.
- Hypoxia due to inadequacies of breathing or circulation will have early effects on the childs level of consciousness.

Assessment of conscious level in the child can be difficult particularly in the pre-verbal child when the traditional Glasgow Coma scale (GCS) may not prove that useful. The modified Children's Glasgow Coma Scale allows the clinician to calculate a more accurate coma scale and should be used in children under the age of 5 (Table 10.4).

Table 10.4 Children's Glasgow Coma Scale

	Time	
Best eye response	Eyes open spontaneously	4
	Eye opening to verbal command.	3
	Eye opening to pain	2
	No eye opening	1
Best verbal response	Smiles, oriented to sounds, follows objects, interacts	5
	Cries but is consolable, inappropriate interactions	4
	Inconsistently consolable, moaning	3
	Inconsolable, agitated	2
	No vocal response	1
Best motor response	Obeys commands	6
	Localising pain	5
	Withdrawal from pain	4
	Flexion to pain	3
	Extension to pain.	2
	No motor response.	1
	Total score	

Box 10.4 AVPU scale

A – Alert (GCS 15)
V – Responds to voice (GCS 13)
P – Responds to pain (GCS 8)
U – Unresponsive (GCS 3)

The use of the AVPU (Alert, Verbal, Pain, Unresponsive) scale detailed in Box 10.4 enables a rapid assessment to be made and may be roughly equated to a GCS.

Pupils and posture should also be evaluated for abnormalities. If there is suspicion of intracranial injury then a CT scan should be performed at the earliest opportunity once the child has been stabilised.

Children are at particular risk of rapidly becoming hypoglycaemic due to their high metabolic rate. Blood glucose should be tested as hypoglycaemia can complicate an already difficult situation. Hypoglycaemic children should receive an IV bolus of 5 ml/kg of 10% dextrose.

Exposure

It is imperative to visualise all of the child and remove all clothing to assess the child for any other injuries, which may be limb or life threatening. Children have a significantly higher body surface area to volume ratio and as a result are prone to losing heat more rapidly than the adult patient. The use of warming blankets can help to reduce heat loss and subsequent hypothermia.

Young children are as aware of their body image as their adolescent counterparts and as a result it is important to respect the child's right to privacy and maintain their modesty as much as is practicably possible.

Log rolling

The paediatric patient will need to be log rolled in order to inspect their back for any injuries, to palpate the length of the spine for any tenderness and to complete the primary survey. The principles of log rolling remain the same but a smaller child will require fewer people to safely log roll.

Babies and infants can be successfully log rolled by two people with one individual taking control of the C-spine and shoulders and the other taking responsibility for the pelvis and legs (Figure 10.4). As the child gets older the number of people required increases until the same process is adopted as for the adult patient.

When log rolling it is important that the examining clinician is the most experienced and most appropriate individual for the task and this is particularly important if rectal examination is required in the suspicion of spinal trauma. This is extremely distressing for any child and as a result it should only be performed once, which is achievable if performed by a competent

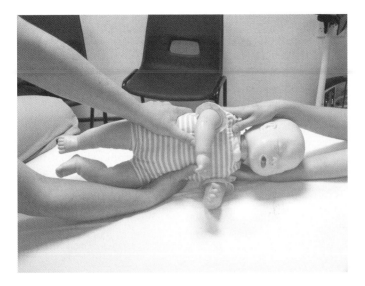

Fig. 10.4 Log rolling an Infant

clinician. Vaginal examination is rarely indicated in children unless there is obvious trauma to the genitals, again this should only be performed once by the most experienced clinician.

Analgesia for injured children

Case study 10.2 Analgesia for injured children

A 10-year-old child has fallen 10 feet from a climbing frame and has a swollen deformed right thigh which paramedics suspect is an isolated fracture of the right femur. The paramedics have been unable to get the child to use inhalation analgesia (nitrous oxide) due to his extreme distress.

On arrival at the ED he is screaming in pain whenever any of the trauma team goes near him. His mother is

---

accompanying him and she is obviously upset at her child's pain.

The trauma team leader and the nurse in charge have to quickly decide which type of analgesia should be given to the child.

The seriously injured child who is conscious is likely to be in a severe amount of pain and analgesia should be administered as soon as possible. Intravenous (IV) morphine is the drug of choice and should be titrated according to the child's pain at a dose of 0.1–0.2 mg/kg.[9] Intramuscular administration is not recommended for children as it is painful and less effective than other methods. Regional nerve blocks may prove more beneficial in some cases and femoral nerve blocks are widely accepted as good practice in the management of femoral fractures.[10]

SECONDARY SURVEY

The principles of the secondary survey in the paediatric patient remain the same as in the adult patient. Once life-threatening injuries have been identified and successful resuscitation completed, the child should be fully examined for any other injuries. This involves the same top to toe, front to back, examination and completion of radiographs as described in Chapter 2, however there are some additional factors that should be considered in caring for the paediatric patient.

Cervical spine clearance and SCIWORA

Cervical spine immobilisation, as described previously, can be difficult in children. However, once successful immobilisation is achieved it is vital that it is continued until the cervical spine can be fully assessed. During assessment manual immobilisation should be maintained as accurate examination is impossible with a rigid collar in place. The child's cervical spine may only be cleared once x-rays and a clinical examination have been completed and found to be normal. This should be performed by an experienced clinician as children may suffer significant damage to their spinal cord and yet have completely normal x-ray images.

Spinal Cord Injury Without Radiological Abnormality (SCIWORA) is very common in children, accounting for 55% of all spinal injuries in children under the age of 8 and as a result radiological and clinical examination must be completed before immobilisation precautions are withdrawn. Conversely a proportion of children, approximately 9% aged 1–7 years, have a normal pseudosubluxation of either C2 on C3 or C3 on C4, where the vertebrae seem to be out of normal alignment, which can make interpretation of images very difficult.[3]

Child protection

Obtaining an accurate history is always vital regardless of age as it can give information, which may be useful in predicting possible injuries or severity. In addition this information should provide the clinician with details such as:

- Pre-existing medical conditions
- Medication history
- The ingestion of any alcohol or drugs
- Immunisation status
- Known allergies.

However, when dealing with the paediatric patient it is vital that the history does not simply address the mechanism of the injury but in addition provides information about how the child came to be in that situation in the first place. For example knowing that a child has fallen out of a second storey window may provide information about the forces involved and potential injury patterns, however it does not identify the factors that lead to the incident occurring. Was there a faulty window? Was the child left unsupervised? Was there a fire in the house and the only method of escape was out of the window? Identification of such factors is important in addressing the possibility of child protection issues and the need for referral to other agencies. Box 10.5 provides prompts in the form of the

---

Box 10.5 CWILTED child protection prompts

CONDITION: Area of pain, problem
WITNESS: Name, position and designation of person who actually saw incident
INCIDENT: Mechanism which caused the injury
Immunisation status
LOCATION: Home address, name of school
TIME: Time of incident, time of first aid (including medication given), time of last meal
ESCORT: Who is with them, do they have parental responsibility, if they were not a witness then how do they know what happened?
DESCRIPTION: What does the child look like?
How are they behaving?

---

mnemonic CWILTED, which has been successfully used in many paediatric units.[11]

Psychological effects of trauma

Children pose a number of interesting difficulties in relation to their cognitive development and its impact on their care. Young children are extremely phobic and a strange environment, surrounded by unfamiliar faces and fear of what might happen to them, may all contribute to an extremely distressed child. It is not possible to bargain with a child until the age of at least 6 as they are unable to understand cause and effect relationships. The use of other techniques to aid compliance such as distraction may be more beneficial in this age group.[12] It is also important to remember that fear, pain and distress may all result in regression and the child may begin to respond in a more immature manner than expected.

The use of bubbles, toys, books or simply talking to the child about their favourite cartoon, toy or friend will help to provide familiarity. If a play specialist is available then they should be included in the management of the paediatric trauma patient from the earliest possibility. There is, however, no substitute for keeping parents or carers close to the child who can help to calm and reassure the child as well as enabling the parent to be reassured by being able to see what is happening to their child. The parent can also help to obtain clinical information from the child, for example identifying the location of any pain, as the child is much more likely to respond to a familiar face and give accurate information.

It is important that the practitioner communicates appropriately with the child and family and keeps the child informed of what is happening. Knowledge helps to allay fear and this will ultimately make clinical assessment easier, however information must be phrased in a way that the child can understand. Play can be a very useful tool and the use of teddy bears or dolls to illustrate to a child what needs to be done can assist in establishing a degree of normality for the child.

CONCLUSION

The priorities in caring for the paediatric patient remain the same as in the adult. Anatomical and physiological differences are reflected in their responses to injury and change with age. Psychological and developmental factors should be considered in their management and a clear history obtained to exclude the possibility of child protection concerns.

KEY INFORMATION BOX

- Treatment priorities of the paediatric patient remain the same as in the adult
- Anatomical and physiological differences in children give rise to varying observations with age
- The most common cause of cardiorespiratory arrest in the paediatric patient is hypoxia, so optimum oxygenation and ventilation is vital
- Child protection concerns must be considered during the management of the traumatised child
- Use of distraction and ensuring parents or carers are near to the child will enable the clinician to gain cooperation from the child.

REFERENCES

1. Department of Trade and Industry (2006) Home and Leisure Accident Report. Stationery Office, London

2. Potier K (2005) Broselow Tape or APLS formula to estimate weight in children, Bestbets ref 64. http:www.bestbets.org/cgi-bin/bets.pl?record=00064

3. Advanced Life Support Group (2005) Advanced paediatric life support: the practical approach (4th edn). BMJ Books/Blackwell Publishing, London

4. American College of Surgeons (2004) Pediatric trauma. In: Advanced trauma life support for doctors. Student course manual (7th edn), 243–262. American College of Surgeons, Chicago

5. Clements R, Steel A, Bates A, MacKenzie R (2007) Cuffed endotracheal tube use in paediatric prehospital intubation: challenging the doctrine, Emergency Medicine Journal 54:57–58

6. Pitt E (2005) Role of flexion/extension radiography in paediatric neck injuries, Bestbets Ref 638. http:www.bestbets.org/cgi-bin/bets.pl?record=00638

7. Macgregor J (2000) Introduction to the anatomy and physiology of children. Routledge, London

8. Chamley C, Carson P, Randall D, Sandwell W (2005) Developmental anatomy and physiology of children: a practical approach. Churchill Livingstone, London

9. British National Formulary for Children (2006) Pharmaceutical Press, London

10. Williams R (2000) Regional anaesthesia worked well for children with femoral shaft fractures, Bestbets Ref: 130. http:www.bestbets.org/cgi-bin/bets.pl?record=0013

11. Willis M (2001) CWILTED. Emergency Nurse 8(9):18–22

12. Glasper A, Richardson J (2005) A textbook of children and young people's nursing. Churchill Livingstone, London

Trauma in Older People 11

Antonia Lynch

INTRODUCTION

The population in the United Kingdom is ageing. In 2001, 16% of the population was aged over 65[1] and this is expected to rise. Although the population rose by 8% from 1971 to 2005, the growth did not occur evenly across all age groups. During this time the proportion of people over 65 grew, however the proportion of people less than 16 years of age fell.[2]

Trauma is a major cause of death in patients aged over 65, the most predominant cause of death being falls,[3-5] closely followed by road traffic accidents.[3] Older people are more likely to die from trauma than younger people. This is as a result of physiological changes due to ageing, having multiple medical problems (co-morbidities) and taking more than four or five medications (poly pharmacy). The complex nature of older patients has led a trauma centre in the United States to modify their guidelines to include age >70 years as a criterion for trauma team activation.[6]

The aim of this chapter is to understand the principles of rapid assessment, resuscitation and stabilisation of the seriously injured older person.

LEARNING OBJECTIVES

By the end of this chapter the reader will be able to:

❏ Define the physiology of ageing
❏ Describe assessment and management priorities in relation to ABCDE

❏ Identify unique types and patterns of injury in the older patient

❏ Identify red flags for abuse of the older person.

PHYSIOLOGY OF AGEING

As a person grows older, many physiological functions change. This can affect the way that disease or injury symptoms are manifested. It can also affect the body's response to many factors such as stress, medication, temperature or blood loss.

A comprehensive overview of the physiological changes associated with ageing and the effects of injury are illustrated in Table 11.1. To improve the older patient's chance of survival, knowledge of the physiology of ageing and the effects of multiple medical problems needs to be integrated into the assessment and resuscitation process.

PRIMARY SURVEY

Airway and cervical spine control

Establishing a patent airway is the primary objective, as for any traumatically injured patient.[7] Cervical spine injury caused by hyperextension during a fall is common in older people.[8] As with all trauma patients the patient's neck should be immobilised until a senior clinician can exclude the presence of an injury. The presence of a kyphosis (curvature of the spine – Figure 11.1) can make this uncomfortable for the older person however the risk of injury means that immobilisation must be carried out. Older people are particularly susceptible to cervical spine injury due to pre-existing osteoporosis and osteoarthritis. These conditions also make interpretation of an x-ray difficult and the patient may require early computerised tomography (CT) scan or magnetic resonance imaging (MRI) to determine the presence and extent of an injury.

Breathing and ventilation

Supplemental oxygen should be given early to avoid hypoxia.

Table 11.1 Physiological changes associated with ageing

Primary survey	System	Pre-existing conditions	Physiological changes	Signs and symptoms	Potential traumatic injuries
Airway and cervical spine control	There are no specific physiological changes specific to older people in relation to the airway C-spine, see musculoskeletal				
Breathing	Respiratory	Chronic obstructive pulmonary disease Asthma Pneumonia Pulmonary oedema Pulmonary embolism Congestive heart failure History of smoking	Non-elastic fibrous tissue Fixed expiratory volume Reduced compliance Reduced vital capacity Reduced alveoli in number and size Reduced peak expiratory flow Increased residual volume Hypoventilation despite normal perfusion Reduced baseline PO_2 Reduced cough reflexes Chest wall stiffness Reduced response to foreign antigen Reduced response to hypoxia or hypercarbia	Increased diaphragmatic breathing Shortness of breath	Increased risk of rib fractures Increased risk of pulmonary contusion Air trapping Atelectasis Increased risk of pneumonia Increased risk of aspiration Increased risk of Adult Respiratory Distress Syndrome (ARDS)

Table 11.1 *Cont'd*

Primary survey	System	Pre-existing conditions	Physiological changes	Signs and symptoms	Potential traumatic injuries
Circulation and haemorrhage control	Cardiovascular	Coronary artery disease Hypertension Congestive heart failure Myocardial infarction Medications (beta blockers, calcium channel blockers, anticoagulants)	Fat and fibrous tissue replaces conductive pathways Heart valves thicken reducing compliance Reduced coronary artery flow Lower maximum heart rate Reduced cardiac output	Dysrhythmias Hypertension Inability to meet increased myocardial oxygen demands Heart rate may not rise due to stressors	Aortic arch disruption Myocardial contusion Aneurysm
	Renal	Renal insufficiency	Reduced number of glomeruli Reduced number of nephrons Reduced renal flow Reduced glomerular filtration rate Reduced bladder capacity Reduced drug metabolism	Reduced urinary output	Acute renal failure Increased risk of fluid/electrolyte imbalance and fluid overload
Disability	Central nervous system	Stroke Dementia Alzheimer's Impaired gait		Confusion Altered mental status	Increased risk of subdural haematoma Brain infarct Closed head injury
Exposure		Defects in thermoregulation	Reduced shivering/reduced sweating		Hypo/hyperthermia

Other related co-morbid conditions				
Gastrointestinal	Reduced calorie intake Reduced glucose tolerance	Reduced calorie requirement Reduced body mass Reduced drug metabolism by liver Reduced gastric emptying Reduced gastric motility Reduced oesophageal sphincter	Oesophageal reflux Bowel dysfunction	Increased risk of bowel injuries Mesenteric infarction
Skin and musculoskeletal	Nutritional deficiency Joint disease Arthritis	Loss of skin tone Reduced sensation Loss of resilient connective tissue Reduced mobility Osteoporosis Spondylosis Kyphosis	Bruising Contusions Skin/wound infections	Tetanus Distal radius fractures Fractured hip C1–C2 fractures from falls at ground level Spinal fractures. Rib fractures
Immunological	Autoimmune dysfunction Coagulopathies	Altered cellular response	Sepsis without pyrexia	
Hepatic			Bruising Bleeding	Contusions Bleeding
Endocrine	Diabetes mellitus Diabetes insipidus Thyroid dysfunction	Decreased insulin response, glucose tolerance and sensitivity to antidiuretic hormone		

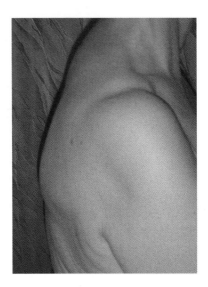

Fig. 11.1 Kyphosis

Ageing reduces lung volume and elasticity whilst calcification of the costal cartilage and rib osteoporosis limits expansion of the rib cage, which results in decreased vital capacity. Respiratory muscle strength is reduced as muscle fibres atrophy, which leaves older people more at risk of respiratory fatigue. Therefore, hypoxia can have a rapid onset. In order to detect problems early, close monitoring of the patient's breathing and ventilation is necessary through systematic assessment of:

- Respiratory rate
- Respiratory depth
- Chest movements
- Work of breathing
- Oxygen saturations.

Patients with chronic obstructive pulmonary disease retain carbon dioxide. These patients lose their normal respiratory drive produced by an elevated PCO_2 and have a hypoxic respiratory drive.[7] However, *regardless of their age*, trauma patients must not remain hypoxic as this may prove fatal and they should be given 15 L/min of oxygen via a non-rebreathe mask. Arterial blood gases should be gained as soon as possible to ensure adequate oxygenation and ventilation is being achieved. If the older patient's respiratory status deteriorates, they may require intubation and full ventilatory support.

Older people are occasionally without teeth (edentulous) and some may have loose fitting dentures, which can make bag-valve-mask ventilation difficult due to poor fitting face-masks. Well fitting dentures should be noted and left in place to aid mask fitting.

Identification of the life-threatening chest injuries is a priority as the mortality rate from these conditions is higher in the older person.[7] These include:

- Tension pneumothorax
- Haemothorax
- Cardiac tamponade.

Rib fractures and chest wall contusions are not deemed imminently life threatening; however, they pose a risk to older people. These injuries are poorly tolerated and may result in sudden deterioration and respiratory failure.[6]

A combination of poor chest wall compliance, pre-existing conditions such as COPD and poor pain control can lead to hypoventilation and, in the long term, infection. Adequate pain control with analgesia such as intravenous morphine is essential. Older patients must be asked directly about their pain, as older people are less likely to report pain.

Circulation and haemorrhage control

Case study 11.1 Cardiovascular assessment in older trauma patients

A 76-year-old female is hit by a car at 30 mph whilst crossing the road. On arrival to the ED she looks very pale

---

> and is obviously in pain. Her initial vital signs are recorded as: RR 25, HR 68, BP 122/76. She tells the doctor that she takes 'blood pressure medicine, aspirin, a heart tablet and a water tablet'.

Cardiovascular assessment is more complex in older patients due to the effects of pre-existing cardiac disease and the effects of poly pharmacy.

When an older person suffers a traumatic injury there is the same release of catecholamines (adrenaline and noradrenaline) in response to blood loss. In a younger person this would cause tachycardia, however some older people have reduced sensitivity to catecholamines and therefore the pulse and other vital signs remain within normal limits.

Poly pharmacy is common among older people.[9] Common medications include:

- Beta-blockers
- Angiotension-converting enzyme (ACE) inhibitors
- Diuretics
- Anticoagulants.

These medications may complicate the patient's response to injury and alter the patient's initial clinical presentation. A 'normal' or 'mildly low' blood pressure in a chronically hypertensive patient may in reality signify severe hypotension.[6] For example an older person whose blood pressure is normally high, e.g. 170/110, will be very hypotensive if their blood pressure falls to 110/70, although this is seen as a 'normal BP'. Similarly, absence of a tachycardia does not rule out hypovolaemia, especially if the patient is taking beta-blockers.

Older people have limited cardiac reserve; therefore a rapid assessment for blood loss should be made. A Focused Assessment with Sonography for Trauma (FAST) examination should be performed to detect the presence of abnormal intra-abdominal fluid. Retroperitoneal bleeding often goes unnoticed and older people are particularly vulnerable to this caused by hip, pelvic or vertebral fractures.[7]

Fluid resuscitation using intravenous crystalloid may be administered according to the patient's vital signs and physiological status (see Chapter 2). Blood transfusions may be needed if the patient is hypovolaemic, to increase delivery of oxygen.

The patient's circulatory status and renal function can be monitored by the insertion of a urinary catheter. The kidney reduces in mass with age and experiences a progressive loss of glomeruli resulting in a loss of function. Therefore, initial urine output may not be a good indicator of perfusion.

Disability and dysfunction

Nurses play a pivotal role in establishing a rapport with trauma patients, endeavouring to reassure them and maintain a safe environment during this time. History regarding the patient's pre-existing mental dysfunction, i.e. Alzheimer's or other dementia, should be gained from relatives, friends or carers at the earliest convenience.

Accurate neurological assessment is required but can be challenging in older people. Physiological changes include:

- Cerebral atrophy (reduction in the size of the brain) occurs during ageing due to a progressive loss of neurons.
- The dura (outer layer of the meninges) becomes adhered to the skull.
- The parasagittal bridging veins can become stretched making them more susceptible to rupture.
- A smaller brain results in increased space within the skull, allowing the brain more space to move about in the skull leaving it vulnerable to injury.
- Large amounts of blood can be lost into the increased space and overt clinical signs can be subtle and delayed in comparison to younger patients.[7]

Older people are three times more likely to suffer from sub-dural haematoma than younger people. There is also an increased incidence of intracerebral haematoma, which may be in part caused by taking anticoagulants.[7]

A Glasgow Coma Scale should be performed to assess the patient's level of consciousness. Anxiety, disorientation and confusion must be assumed to be as a result of injury and should be treated as for any trauma patient rather than assuming it is the patient's' normal mental state.[10] If a head injury is suspected, the management is the same for all trauma patients and an early CT scan is recommended.

Exposure and environment control

A log roll is required to ensure the patient's back is inspected for injury. Older patients may have a fear of falling when being rolled and careful explanation is required.

Skin and connective tissue alters during the ageing process, this includes loss of strength, vascularity and function. During ageing the epidermis takes longer to regenerate and the dermis loses up to 20% of its thickness.[7] These changes affect the older person's ability to regulate temperature. Also, skin tears easily which leaves it vulnerable to trauma and wound healing is impaired. Surgical scars may give an indication to the patient's past medical history. It should be recognised that even small wounds can be a potential source of bacterial infection and should be assessed and irrigated thoroughly. Enquiry into the patient's tetanus immunisation status is required and a booster prescribed and administered if needed (see Chapter 2).

To visualise and inspect all potential injuries, the patient must be fully undressed. Older patients are vulnerable to hypothermia and should not be left uncovered for any length of time. Patient's privacy and dignity remain important, it is the role of the team to ensure patients are not left exposed after the initial inspection, however, nurses often have greater awareness of this.

SECONDARY SURVEY

This is the top to toe examination of the patients, to detect and assess those injuries which are not life threatening.

Patients may remain immobilised for long periods of time and consideration should be given to pressure areas when the patient is stabilised. Patients must not be left lying on spinal boards. Older patients are less likely to report pain from pressure points due to reduced pain receptors.

Abuse of the older person

Have a high index of suspicion if the history is inconsistent with the injury pattern.

The prevalence of abuse of the older person in the UK is relatively unknown. Abuse often goes unreported by the patient and unnoticed by healthcare professionals due to failure to recognise 'red flags' displayed by patients and/or their abusers. Patients may present with life-threatening trauma as a result of abuse or this may be detected as part of the secondary survey.

Nurses should have a high index of suspicion when assessing older people, as with non-accidental injury in children. Clinicians must assess whether the mechanism is consistent with the injury or illness presented.[11] All staff need to be aware of the red flags of abuse, as illustrated in Box 11.1,[12,13] and the appropriate action to be taken in cases of suspected abuse. If abuse of the older person is suspected:

- Attention to detail when documenting is of paramount importance
- Document the person's account in their own words[14] and signs of abuse clearly
- Consider the use of illustration through medical photography, which requires specialist consent and adherence to local guidelines
- Upon detection of abuse, local guidelines should be adhered to in relation to reporting to police, social services, etc.

Box 11.1 The red flags for abuse of the older person[13,14]

Signs of physical abuse:

- Multiple bruising, e.g. inner thigh or bruising at different stages of healing
- Finger marks
- Burns, especially in unusual places
- An injury similar to the shape of an object
- Unexplained fractures
- Pressure ulcers or untreated wounds
- Attempts to hide part of the body on examination
- Inappropriate use of medications, e.g. overdosing

Signs of sexual abuse:

- Pain, itching or injury to the anal, genital or abdominal area
- Difficulty in walking or sitting because of genital pain
- Bruising and/or bleeding of external genitalia
- Torn, stained or bloody underclothes
- Sexually transmitted disease or recurrent episodes of cystitis
- An uncharacteristic change in the patients attitude to sex
- Unexplained problems with catheters

Signs of neglect:

- Weight loss
- Unkempt appearance, dirty clothes and poor hygiene
- Pressure ulcers or uncharacteristic problems with continence
- Inadequate nutrition and hydration
- Inadequate or inappropriate medical treatment or withholding treatment
- A patient who is left in a wet or soiled bed

Signs of psychological abuse:

The patient –
- Appears depressed, frightened, withdrawn, apathetic, anxious or aggressive
- Makes a great effort to please

- Appears afraid of being treated by specific staff, carer or relative
- Displays reluctance to be discharged
- Demonstrates sudden mood or behaviour change

CONCLUSION

Older people have higher mortality rates from trauma; they require the application of the same principles of practice. However, the nurse must have the specialist knowledge of the physiology of ageing and apply this to the management of trauma if patient outcomes are to be optimised.

KEY INFORMATION BOX

- Older trauma patients should receive 15 L/min of oxygen via a non-rebreathe mask despite a diagnosis of chronic obstructive pulmonary disease (COPD)
- Rib fractures and chest wall contusions are poorly tolerated in older people and they may deteriorate suddenly
- Absence of a tachycardia in older people does not rule out hypovolaemia
- If you suspect an older patient may have been a victim of abuse, report this to the trauma team leader or the senior nurse.

REFERENCES

1. ONS (2007) The census in England and Wales. http://www.statistics.gov.uk/census2001
2. ONS (2007) Ageing. http://www.statistics.gov.uk/cci/nugget.asp?id=949
3. ONS (2004) Deaths by age, sex and underlying cause http://www.statistics.gov.uk/STATBASE/Expodata/spreadsheets/D8986.xls
4. Department of Health (2001) National Service Framework for older people. Department of Health, London

5. Aminzadeh F, Dalziel WB (2002) Older adults in the emergency department: a systematic review of patterns of use, adverse outcomes and effective interventions. Annals of Emergency Medicine 39:238–247

6. Demetriades D, Sava JMD, Alo K, Newton E, Velmahos GC, Murray JA, Belzberg H, Asensio JA, Berne TV (2001) Old age as a criterion for trauma team activation. Journal of Trauma, Injury, Infection and Critical Care 51:754–757

7. American College of Surgeons (2004) Trauma in the elderly. In: Advanced trauma life support for doctors. Student course manual (7th edn), 263–273. American College of Surgeons, Chicago

8. Lovasik K (1999) The older patient with a spinal cord injury. Critical Care Nursing Quarterly 22(2):20–23

9. Department of Health (2001) National Service Framework for older people. Medicines and older people, implementing medicines-related aspects of the NSF for older people. Department of Health, London

10. Gwinnutt C, Driscoll P (2003) Trauma resuscitation: the team approach (2nd edn). BIOS Scientific Publishers, Oxford

11. Crouch R (2003) Emergency care of the older person. In: Emergency nursing care, principles and practice (Eds Jones G, Endacott R, Crouch R), 75–90. GMM, London

12. Klein Schmidt KC (1997) Elder abuse: a review. Annals of Emergency Medicine 30:463–472

13. Action on Elder Abuse (2005) Indicators of abuse. www.elderabuse.org.uk

14. Community and District Nursing Association (2003) Responding to elder abuse. CDNA, London

Trauma in Pregnancy

12

Antonia Lynch

INTRODUCTION

Trauma involving a pregnant female is relatively rare, however maternal death is most frequently caused by road traffic accidents (RTAs) and domestic violence.[1] Between 2000 and 2002 there were seven maternal deaths as a result of RTAs, of these, two women died from uterine rupture. In addition, 11 women were murdered by their partner and 43 reported domestic violence during pregnancy to a healthcare professional.[1]

The overarching focus in caring for the pregnant trauma patient is *save the mother to save the baby.* A multidisciplinary approach is the best way to optimise both the mother and the foetus' chance of survival. The trauma team needs to include a senior obstetrician and neonatologist to ensure that expert help is available.

The aim of this chapter is to understand the principles of the rapid assessment, resuscitation and stabilisation of the seriously injured pregnant patient.

LEARNING OBJECTIVES

At the end of this chapter the reader will be able to:

❏ Define anatomical and physiological changes during pregnancy
❏ Describe assessment and management priorities for mother and foetus in relation to ABCDE
❏ Identify unique types and patterns of injury in the pregnant patient
❏ Identify red flags for domestic violence.

ANATOMICAL AND PHYSIOLOGICAL CHANGES IN PREGNANCY

The priorities for assessment and management of the traumatically injured pregnant woman follow the same principles as for any trauma patient. However, these priorities may have to be adapted due to anatomical and physiological changes during pregnancy, as illustrated in Table 12.1. These changes in care will differ depending on the stage of pregnancy. There are three trimesters during pregnancy:

- The first exists until the 12th week
- The second from the 13th to the 28th week
- The third spans from the 29th to the 40th week.

Table 12.1 Anatomical and physiological changes in pregnancy

System/organ	Changes relevant to trauma
Uterus	First trimester: intrapelvic until 12th week Second trimester: intra-abdominal. Foetus protected by amniotic fluid Third trimester: uterus is large and thin walled making it more vulnerable to injury
Cardiovascular system	Increased plasma volume and decreased vascular resistance of uterus and placenta cause increased cardiac output Increased cardiac rate Second trimester: decrease in systolic and diastolic blood pressure
Respiratory system	Increased minute volume and tidal volume Third trimester: hypocapnia Decreased residual volume
Haematological	Plasma volume increases until week 34 Increase in red blood cells, decreasing haematocrit May lose 1200–1500 ml of blood volume before displaying signs and symptom of hypovolaemia
Gastro-intestinal system	Gastric emptying time is prolonged Third trimester: bowel lies mostly in upper abdomen Position of liver and spleen remain unchanged
Other systems	Dilation of the renal calyces, pelvis and ureters The symphysis pubis and sacroiliac joints widen

Uterus

The uterus remains in the pelvic cavity until approximately the 12th week when it rises to the abdomen. It reaches the umbilicus by the 20th week and the costal margins of the ribs by weeks 30–34.[2] In the second trimester the foetus is cushioned by large amounts of amniotic fluid but by the third trimester the uterus is large and thin walled.[3] As a result the foetus and placenta have an increased susceptibility to trauma during this trimester. In the last two weeks of pregnancy, the foetus engages, pushing its head down into the pelvis. If the mother sustains a pelvic fracture the foetus is at risk of skull fractures and intracranial injury.[2]

Cardiovascular system

Increases in cardiac output and blood volume begin early in the first trimester and are 30–40% higher than the non-pregnant state by 28 weeks.[4] This allows adequate perfusion for both the mother and the foetus and allows for normal blood loss during labour. As a result of this, the pregnant trauma patient can lose 30–35% of blood before displaying signs and symptoms of hypovolaemia. Maternal blood flow is maintained at the expense of the foetus, as the body will shunt blood from the non-vital organs, such as the uterus.[5] *As a result, by the time the mother displays signs and symptoms of hypovolaemia the foetus will already be in distress.*

The cardiac output increases 1.0–1.5 L/min after the 10th week of pregnancy due to an increase in blood volume and a decrease in vascular resistance of the uterus and placenta.[6] Blood pressure in the first and second trimester is therefore lower due to vasodilation, it then returns to the pre-pregnancy baseline in the third trimester.

Maternal blood pressure and cardiac output are sensitive to maternal position and lying flat on the back – the supine position should be avoided in pregnancy.[6] The enlarged uterus can compress the vena cava reducing venous return to the heart, which decreases cardiac output and causes the blood pressure to drop.

Heart rate increases by 10–15 beats/min in pregnancy, reaching a maximum in the third trimester. This should be taken into consideration when interpreting vital signs of a traumatised pregnant woman.

Respiratory system
There are some anatomical changes that help maintain lung volume and adequate oxygenation to the mother and foetus during pregnancy:

- The diaphragm elevates causing the lungs to decrease in length and increase intrathoracic pressure.
- The rib cage flares out to compensate for the shortening lung length.[5]
- Maternal oxygen consumption is increased during pregnancy; therefore it is important to ensure arterial oxygenation is maintained during resuscitation.[2]
- Minute ventilation (the volume of air inhaled and exhaled each minute) increases.
- Tidal volume (the volume of air inhaled each breath) increases by 40%, caused by increased levels of progesterone.
- Respirations may appear deeper and faster than in a non-pregnant person. This 'hyperventilation' results in lower than normal CO_2 level (or hypocapnia) with a $PaCO_2$ of 30 mmHg.[6]

Haematological changes
Pregnancy causes an increased plasma volume of 20–30% resulting in a decreased haemoglobin and haematocrit. This is known as physiological anaemia. The white blood cell count increases during pregnancy from 12,000 to 25,000 mm^3 in response to stress and, later, labour. Serum fibrinogen and other clotting factors are mildly elevated. Clotting times are shorter and the pregnant patient's blood can clot more quickly. This places the pregnant patient at risk of developing thromboemboli and disseminated intravascular coagulation (DIC).[5]

Gastro-intestinal

The effects of the hormone progesterone on the smooth muscle cause a decrease in gastro-oesophageal sphincter control, an increase in gastric acid secretions and a decrease in stomach emptying, which result in reflux.

To avoid aspiration of food from the stomach into the lungs, the trauma team should always assume the patient's stomach is full, despite the time of their last meal. To assist in stomach emptying a gastric tube should be inserted early.

Urinary

The glomerular filtration rate and renal blood flow both increase in pregnancy. Glycosuria is common in pregnancy. Urine output increases throughout pregnancy with greater excretion of creatinine and urea. As a result, serum creatinine and urea levels may only be half of the pre-pregnancy level.

Musculoskeletal

The symphysis pubis and the sacroiliac joints widen during pregnancy by 4–8 mm, this should be taken into consideration when interpreting pelvic x-rays.[2]

Neurological

A pregnant patient who has had a head injury may present with vague symptoms of headache, drowsiness, visual distur- bances or seizures. However, these symptoms may also be due to pre-eclampsia or eclampsia, and advice from an obstetri- cian should be obtained urgently.

ASSESSMENT AND RESUSCITATION OF THE PREGNANT WOMAN

Primary survey

Airway and cervical spine control
Ensure the patient has a patent airway and cervical spine control.

If there is any suspicion of airway problems with a pregnant woman, an experienced anaesthetist should be called early. Capillaries in the upper airways become engorged in pregnancy which leads to increased soft tissue bulk of the larynx and narrowing of the airways. This, accompanied with breast enlargement and fat deposition on the face, can make intubation difficult.[6]

Breathing and ventilation
Supplemental oxygen, 15 L/min via a non-rebreath mask, is essential to prevent maternal and foetal hypoxia.

As described earlier, minute volume and tidal volume increase with a small increase in respiration rate. A greatly increased respiration rate is a cause for concern as it may be due to lung injury or hypovolaemic shock.

Circulation and haemorrhage control
To prevent vena cava compression, pregnant patients beyond 20 weeks' gestation should not be left lying flat on

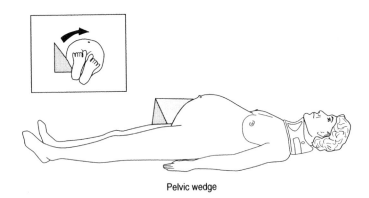

Pelvic wedge

Fig. 12.1 Pelvic wedge in situ to displace the uterus. (Reproduced with permission from Hodgetts T, Turner L (2006) Trauma rules 2 (2nd edn), figure 39.1. Blackwell Publishing, Oxford)

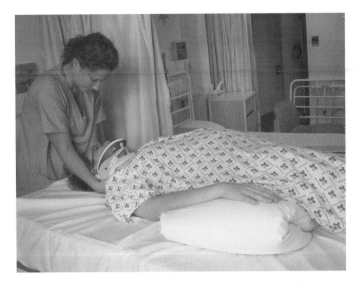

Fig. 12.2 Cervical spine immobilisation for the pregnant patient with a wedge in situ

their back or supine.[4] The patient should be moved into the left lateral position as soon as possible. If the patient is not on a spinal board, a wedge or folded pillow can be placed under the mother's right hip to displace the uterus off the vena cava (Figure 12.1). Cervical spine immobilisation can continue during this position change (Figure 12.2). If a wedge or pillow are not available, the uterus can be displaced manually, i.e. pulling the uterus over to the left.

Severe trauma stimulates maternal catecholamine release, adrenaline and noradrenaline, which causes tachycardia and vasoconstriction. Foetal circulation may be compromised as vasoconstriction also occurs in the uterus and placenta.

Case study 12.1 Altered vital signs in pregnancy

A 27-year-old woman who is 38 weeks pregnant is brought to the ED. She was a front seat restrained passenger during an RTA. The car she was sitting in was hit on the left hand side by a fast moving lorry. On admission to the ED she is pale and distressed. The left hand side of her chest is badly contused and she is struggling to breathe. She also has left abdominal abrasions and the nurse undressing her notes fresh red blood coming from her vagina.

Despite these injuries, her pulse and blood pressure seem to be within normal limits for a woman of her age.

Due to the increase in intravascular volume, pregnant patients can have significant blood loss before displaying a tachycardia or hypotension. The foetus may be in distress, not receiving enough blood from the mother, while the mother's vital signs appear normal.[2] Aggressive fluid resuscitation with crystalloid fluids or type specific blood is indicated to support the physiological hypervolaemia of pregnancy. A surgeon and an obstetrician should be called immediately.

Diagnostic imaging such as a FAST scan may help to identify where the patient is bleeding. If a DPL is performed (see Chapter 2), the catheter should be inserted above the umbilicus.[2]

If chest or pelvic injuries are suspected, x-rays or CT scans should be performed on the pregnant patient as the benefits outweigh the potential risk to the foetus.[2]

Disability and dysfunction
The pregnant patient's neurological state should be assessed in the same way as any trauma patient. Monitoring of the patient's level of consciousness using the GCS should be carried out. Pre-eclampsia can present with a reduced level of consciousness and symptoms similar to a head injury.

Exposure and environment control
The patient should have all clothing removed to ensure that no injuries are missed but care should be taken to avoid uncontrolled hypothermia.

Secondary survey

As with all trauma patients, this is a systematic head to toe and anterior/posterior inspection and examination to detect further injury. A full obstetric history should be taken and foetal assessment should be carried out by an obstetrician.

If the patient is awake and able to talk, useful obstetric information can be gained by asking:

- The date of last menstrual period
- The expected date of delivery
- If there are any complications with current or previous pregnancies.

Specific pregnancy related maternal assessment
Assessment of the pregnant patient must include:

- Measuring the fundal height in centimetres (cm) from the symphysis pubis can determine uterine size. This provides a rapid measure of foetal age; 1 cm equals 1 week gestational age.[8]
- Inspection and examination of the abdomen should detect presence of foetal movement, uterine contractions and tenderness.
- A pelvic examination should be performed to rule out vaginal bleeding or amniotic fluid, ruptured membranes, a bulging perineum and the presence of contractions.[4]

Causes for concern include:

- The presence of uterine contractions suggestive of early labour, or separation of the placenta.[2]
- A change in shape may signify uterine rupture or concealed bleeding.[6]

- The presence of amniotic fluid from the vagina can be evidenced by a pH of 7–7.5 (normal vaginal pH = 5) and suggests ruptured amniotic membranes.
- Vaginal bleeding in the third trimester may indicate disruption of the placenta and impending death of the foetus.[2]

Specific pregnancy related foetal assessment

Foetal assessment should be carried out following maternal resuscitation by an obstetrician, as the foetus is potentially viable beyond 24 weeks. This assessment must include:

- Assessment of the foetal heart rate by auscultation, a doppler or ultra sound if the equipment and expertise is available in the emergency room. The normal foetal heart should range from 120 to 160 beats per minute; bradycardia is a sign that the foetus is in distress. Continuous electronic foetal heart rate monitoring (EFM) is the most widely used modality for foetal evaluation; this is also an adjunct for monitoring the mother's condition.[4]

Specific problems for the traumatised pregnant patient

If any of the following problems are suspected or detected, obstetric help should be sought immediately:

Premature labour

This can be caused by traumatic injury and is easier to note in the awake patient who may experience backache, contractions or vaginal discharge that may be clear or bloody. A vaginal examination may reveal a dilated cervix, indicating the onset of labour.

Uterine rupture

This is a rare complication of blunt abdominal trauma, however this event can be catastrophic for the mother and foetus. The signs that the uterus has ruptured include abdominal pain, tender uterus, vaginal bleeding and signs of maternal hypovolaemic shock.

Placental abruption

This is caused by blunt trauma especially following RTAs.[6] It occurs in 40–50% of pregnant patients with major traumatic injuries[7] and it can cause maternal and foetal death. The uterus consists of a significant proportion of elastic fibres; in comparison, the placenta is mainly inelastic.[3] Placental abruption occurs when the placenta shears from the wall of the uterus causing haemorrhage. Clinical signs include:

- Vaginal bleeding
- Uterine tenderness
- Premature labour
- Abdominal cramps.

Penetrating trauma

The foetus is at risk of penetrating injury to the abdomen, chest or back, as it sits in the abdominal cavity. Maternal survival is usually good if bleeding is controlled, as the uterus is a non-vital organ. However, foetal death is common if the penetrating object enters the foetus.

Emergency caesarean section

If the mother is cardiovascularly stable following traumatic injury but there is concern about the foetus, a caesarean section may be performed as an emergency.

If the mother is in cardiopulmonary arrest due to hypovolaemia following traumatic injury there is little evidence to support a caesarean section, as the outcome is invariably poor. The foetus will have suffered prolonged hypoxia.

DOMESTIC VIOLENCE AND THE PREGNANT TRAUMA PATIENT

Case study 12.2 Recognition of domestic violence

A 22-year-old woman is brought to the ED by her partner. She is 29 weeks pregnant and states that she has tripped

---

and fallen down a flight of stairs at home. She is complaining of lower back and abdominal pain. The nurse notes from the ED records that this is her third attendance in the past 2 months. Whilst helping the patient to get undressed, the nurse notices old bruising on her breasts and abdomen. When questioned about it, the patient is quiet and seems reluctant to comment. Her partner says that she is very clumsy, especially as she is getting bigger, and that 'she's always tripping over'.

Domestic violence is an increasing cause of maternal trauma and clinicians need to have knowledge of the red flags for domestic violence (Box 12.1). If suspected, it is important to ask the patient directly without the presence of the partner and seek senior advice.

Box 12.1 Red flags for domestic violence

The following should be noted in all pregnant trauma patients:

- Late booking of pregnancy to obstetric services
- Repeat attendances to emergency department/GP/walk-in centres/minor injury units with minor injuries
- Signs and symptoms inconsistent with history
- Injuries to head, neck, breasts, abdomen and genital area
- Repeat presentation with anxiety, depression, self harm
- The woman appearing evasive or reluctant to speak especially in front of partner
- Constant presence of the partner at examinations, may answer all the questions and be unwilling to leave the room
- Poor obstetric history
- Recurrent sexually transmitted diseases
- Unexplained hospital admissions

CONCLUSION

The principles of assessment and management for the pregnant trauma patient follow those of the non-pregnant patients; however, pregnant women require special consideration. Clinicians must have an awareness of the anatomical and physiological changes relating to pregnancy to optimise survival. Mothers may have significant blood loss without a change in vital signs during which time the foetus will be experiencing hypoxia. The most effective way to optimise foetal survival is to optimise maternal resuscitation.

KEY INFORMATION BOX

- Intubation may be difficult and an experienced anaesthetist should be involved early
- Respiratory rate may be increased due to pregnancy, however be suspicious if it is greatly raised
- Log roll the pregnant patient into the left lateral position; use a pillow if a wedge is unavailable
- Pregnant patients can have significant blood loss before displaying a tachycardia or hypotension
- Domestic violence is a common cause of injury in pregnant women.

REFERENCES

1. Why mothers die (2000–2002) Confidential Enquiry into Maternal and Child Health. www.cemach.org.uk/publications.htm
2. American College of Surgeons (2004) Trauma in women. In: Advanced trauma life support for doctors. Student course manual (7th edn), 275–282. American College of Surgeons, Chicago
3. Weintraub AY, Leron E, Mazor M (2006) The pathophysiology of trauma in pregnancy: a review. Journal of Maternal-Fetal and Neonatal Medicine 19:601–605

4. Desjardins G (2003) Management of the injured pregnant patient.   http:www.trauma.org/resus/pregnancytrauma. html

5. D'Amico C (2002) Trauma in pregnancy. Topics in Emergency Medicine 24(4):26–39

6. Fletcher S, Lomas G (2003) Trauma in pregnancy. In: Trauma resuscitation: the team approach (2nd edn) (Eds Gwinnutt C, Driscoll P), 243–252. BIOS Scientific Publishers, Oxford

7. Bridgeman P (2004) Management of pregnant trauma patients. Emergency Nurse 12(5):22–25

8. Tinkoff G (2002) Care of the pregnant trauma patient. In: The trauma manual (2nd ed) (Eds Peitzman AB, Rhodes M, Schwab CW, Yealy DM, Fabian TC), 461–468. Lippincott Williams & Wilkins, Philadelphia

Trauma-related Deaths

13

Sandi Meisner

INTRODUCTION

In England and Wales in 2006 there were 241 fatal injuries at work,[1] 755 homicides (United Kingdom)[2] and 3172 people were killed on the road.[3] Other causes of trauma-related deaths include falls, exposure to fire, heat, intentional self harm and poisoning. These deaths do not all happen in the emergency department (ED) but sometimes much further down the continuum of care and indeed sometimes years after the initial insult. All these deaths will come under some medicolegal investigation, through the coroner's court, civil courts and/or the criminal courts, irrespective of when or where the injury or incident leading to the death occurred. In 2006 Coroners in England and Wales held 29,327 Inquests.[4] Inquiries into all trauma deaths also ensure public safety by identifying circumstances where deaths can be prevented in the future.

The circumstances of the incident leading to the death will not always be known when ED staff are involved in the care and cases do not come to court for sometimes as long as 3 years, therefore it is essential that healthcare professionals (HCP) understand the requirements of the agencies involved in managing death processes. Sudden traumatic death also has an effect on the family and society, therefore how these deaths are managed in the ED can make a difference to the grieving process of bereaved people.

LEARNING OBJECTIVES

At the end of this chapter the reader will be able to:

❏ Identify the agencies involved following a trauma-related death

- ❏ Discuss the role of the coroners service
- ❏ Discuss the role of the police service
- ❏ Identify what could be considered evidence
- ❏ Discuss the preservation of evidence
- ❏ Understand procedures in organ and tissue donation
- ❏ Discuss communication with bereaved people.

THE CORONER

In England and Wales the coroner is an independent judicial officer who, by law, must inquire into certain deaths.[5] Section 8 of the Coroners Act 1988 as amended by section 17A concerns the duty of the coroner to hold an inquest in specific circumstances:

- 8(1) where a coroner is informed that the body of a person is lying within his district and there is reasonable cause to suspect that the deceased:
  - has died a violent or unnatural death;
  - has died a sudden death of which the cause is unknown; or
  - has died in prison or in such a place or in such circumstances as to require an inquest under any other Act

There is a similar system in Northern Ireland. In Scotland the Procurator Fiscal undertakes the inquiries but there are no inquests held in public, however in certain circumstances a Fatal Accident Inquiry is held in the Sheriffs court with the Procurator Fiscal leading the evidence.

- Coroner's work within territorial boundaries or jurisdictions and are usually assisted by coroner's officers.
- *All trauma-related deaths should be reported to the coroner* in whose jurisdiction the body lies irrespective of where or when the injury leading to the death occurred.
- The coroner *may* order a post-mortem examination to establish the cause of death and he/she does not need family consent to do this.
- An inquest is usually opened and then adjourned to allow for inquiries to be made.

- Usually the body of the deceased is released to the entitled person for a funeral before the resumption of the inquest.
- As these deaths are not natural the coroner will inquire into the death by way of an inquest and will either sit by himself or with a jury.
- The coroner's inquest is inquisitorial and not blame apportioning and seeks to establish who the deceased was and how, when and where the deceased came by his/her death.
- Coroners must also record the particulars necessary for a death to be registered (as required by the Registration Act 1953).

Reporting deaths to the coroner

There is no statutory duty for medical or nursing staff in the ED to report a death to the coroner, as this is the responsibility of the Registrar of Deaths. However, to ensure that timely inquiries can be made, that the appropriate agencies are informed and that families are kept informed it is considered best practice for deaths in the ED to be reported.[6] Therefore the ED should establish clear reporting protocols to ensure timely and appropriate information is passed to the coroner or the coroner's officer and that family are kept informed of these processes. Local policy and protocols should be developed in conjunction with and acceptable to the coroner, the police service, the ED and the hospital trust.

Who should report the death?

This will rely on local policy and protocols developed in conjunction with the coroner but would usually be:

- Bereavement services personnel in some circumstances. However, they may not be able to interpret the records or understand the implications of confidentiality.
- Any registered nurse or doctor. They can interpret the records and understand confidentiality but may not have been on duty.
- Ideally the doctor or nurse in charge of the care.

When should the death be reported?

This will rely on local policy and protocols developed in conjunction with the coroner and would usually be by telephone:

- Immediately if police are present and consider the death unexplained or if ED senior staff consider the death to be unexplained (suspicion of a crime).
- The next morning if the death is from traumatic injuries but no suspicion of crime.
- Some coroners may ask to be informed when any deaths occurs in the ED no matter what time of day.

What should be reported?

All details that are known and written on the medical record and requested by the coroner or coroner's office including:

- Name, as known at the time and any other names they are known by
- Date of birth
- Address
- Family or next of kin name and contact details
- General practitioner
- Time of arrival in the ED and by what means?
- Ambulance service details, call sign and contact name/s
- All investigations, procedures, treatments and movement in the ED
- All staff members present *including* the treating doctor
- Doctor who confirms death (sometimes referred to as 'pronouncing life extinct'). *This should not be confused with the doctor who 'certifies' the death – this is the doctor who issues the medical certificate of the cause of death*
- Time of death
- Any other information available at the time which could assist the coroner's inquiries should be disclosed voluntarily and not only when requested[7]
- Any information requested by the coroner or coroner's officer.

Care of property

This will rely on local policy and protocols developed in conjunction with the coroner and police service. Property includes all clothing, the contents of all bags accompanying the patient and pockets and wallets:

- If the patient is unable to care for the property themselves then the ED staff and the hospital should assume control and responsibility for it
- May be taken by the police as evidence
- May be required by the coroner to assist with identification
- *No clothing or property should be given to next of kin or family in the ED unless it is established that neither the police nor the coroner requires it.* This should be explained to the family and they should be reassured that the police or the coroner will discuss this with them if necessary
- Valuables on the body (all jewellery including piercings) should stay on the body but should be taped and documented on the property sheet
- Other valuables including money should be cared for as per the department protocols
- Valuables should only be released to the executor of the will or personal representative if they are in possession of a grant of probate or letters of administration relating to the estate. *It is unlikely that ED staff would be in a position to establish who is entitled to this property and the trust/hospital could be held responsible for handing property to the wrong person.*

Care of the body

At all times the body must be treated with care and respect. The coroner and the police will rely on HCPs not to interfere with the body other than those procedures necessary to prepare the body for transport to a mortuary:

- All IV lines, cut down lines, chest drains and endotracheal tubes should remain in situ. The larger appliances such as external fixators can be removed but this should be documented in the records.

- Clothing on the body at the time of death should be left on the body.
- *No part of the body should be washed or cleaned or interfered with in any way.*
- Any wounds present should be covered with clean dry dressings and should not be cleaned or washed.
- The body should be labelled and placed in a body bag (as per department protocols) to be transported to the hospital or public mortuary.
- Viewing by family members can be facilitated and they should be informed of the presence of blood, on the body, and any apparatus/appliances and the reason for them. The HCP should discuss this with police if present or the coroner's office and the names of those present and the time and place of viewing documented.
- Family members can usually touch the body but some religious or cultural rituals *should be* discouraged if it will interfere with evidence preservation (e.g. washing). This should also be discussed with police if present or the coroner's office.
- A police officer and/or a coroner's officer may accompany the family to the viewing.

Medical records

A copy of the complete medical record, test results and x-rays should be made available to the coroner if requested. This not only assists the coroner in his/her investigation but also the pathologist in determining a cause of death.

Attending a coroner's inquest

A HCP may be requested to attend a coroner's inquest as a witness of fact, either through a simple telephone call, a letter or, more formally, by a witness summons. The summons compels attendance at court and there is a penalty of a fine or imprisonment if there is failure to attend. *The HCP should check they understand why they are being asked to attend*, ensure the date, time and place of the inquest are clear and if necessary ask for written directions.

At the inquest

Inquests are usually held in 'public', the court is open and any member of the public including the media can attend. All witnesses sit in the court during procedures unless the coroner decides otherwise, and the HCP should be aware that they will be first of all asked questions by the coroner and then by other witnesses, considered 'properly interested persons' (the coroner determines who this will be) including the family. Each witness is asked to take an oath or affirmation prior to giving evidence.

The HCP as a witness on the day of the inquest

- Ensure they arrive in good time and are dressed smartly and conservatively.
- Inform the coroner's officer or court usher that they have arrived and follow their guidance on where they should go.
- Have a copy of their report, and ensure the full medical records, including x-rays are available in court if necessary.
- Address the coroner as Sir or Madam.
- The HCP gives evidence as a witness of fact but may be asked to give a professional opinion, if so then the HCP should stay within their area of expertise.
- If asked a question that is considered a breach of confidentiality and would not normally be divulged then inform the coroner. The coroner may direct the HCP to divulge the information requested and then the HCP is protected by due process of the law. A witness could be held to be in contempt of court if they refuse to answer.
- If asked a question that is not understood then ask for clarification.

- A witness will be asked to stand down when their evidence is completed.
- The inquest is concluded when a verdict is given by a jury or the coroner.
- Some courts have a coroner's court support service. These are volunteers who support family and witnesses attending an inquest. They may assist the HCP in explaining the court layout and what procedures to expect.

THE POLICE SERVICE

A police service is a public authority and has a duty to keep communities safe by enforcing the law and investigating crime. Therefore when someone dies from traumatic injuries it is not unusual for police officers to attend the ED and request assistance in the investigation process. To ensure all evidence that is available is protected a police officer may accompany the injured to the hospital to ensure continuity, collect or seize evidence (e.g. clothing) and to consider what forensic opportunities may be lost during the resuscitation process and procedures. They must also try to establish the identity of the person and may request information to assist this process. They will also want to establish a prognosis of the condition of the injured and therefore will want to speak to a member of the medical or nursing team.

Confidentiality and disclosure to a police officer

The HCP should understand that breaching confidentiality puts them at risk to legal challenges from patients, employers and professional regulatory bodies[8] and this includes disclosure to a police officer. The HCP should consult with senior staff and follow the guidelines of the professional bodies, the department protocols, the employers legal department, and if necessary, refer to the Caldecott guardian (usually a senior member of the management board or a board level clinician) of the trust.[9]

Before any information is given to the police, the HCP should establish:

- Who is the right person to do this
- The person is sure of the facts
- That what is said will be written down and the HCP may be called upon in the future to justify any comments.

Police officers may request access to medical records, notes or to attendance records. They can seek an order from a judge for disclosure of medical records under Police and Criminal Evidence Act 1984 (schedule 1). It is unlikely that the police will have this order when the patient is in the ED, therefore access should be denied and this should be documented in the records. *Family members can not consent 'for the patient'*:

- The police do not automatically have a right to see or receive a copy of the medical records.
- Police officers cannot ask to be informed if someone is leaving the department, or ask for them to be detained.

There are exceptions where disclosure of information is required by law and statutes affect all citizens not just HCPs:

- Following a road traffic collision the Road Traffic Act 1991 requires any person to provide the police, when requested, with information which may identify the *vehicle driver/s* involved in an incident. The HCP however must be sure of the facts as it is not always clear in the ED who is the driver.
- Under the Prevention of Terrorism Act 2000 any person who believes a person may have been involved in a terrorist act and has information to support this belief should inform the police.
- A court may order disclosure of information. The HCP can offer an objection on the grounds of confidentiality but if further requested to divulge the information then it should be given.

Public interest disclosure
The Nursing Midwifery Council (NMC) or General Medical Council (GMC) cannot tell HCPs whether to disclose or

withhold information but they, along with the British Medical Association, provide guidance.[10] Public interest is ultimately decided by the courts but the NMC, and the GMC can also require justification of HCP's actions, therefore all decisions should be documented and justifiable.

Firearm wounds

There is no statutory duty to report to the police the presence in the ED of a patient suffering this type of injury. However the Association of Chief Police Officers (ACPO) and GMC[11] have issued guidelines, which require the treating doctor to notify police of patients with firearm wounds. This not only ensures safety of the injured, hospital staff, others in the department and hospital but also the public:

- The treating doctor can delegate this to another staff member.
- Disclosure of name and address should be withheld at this stage.
- Police will ask to speak to the patient; this should not compromise care and remains the treating doctors' decision. The patient, if able, should also give consent. Decisions should be documented.
- If there is any doubt as to whether there should be disclosure then advice should be sought from the treating consultant or the trust's Caldicott guardian.
- *Disclosure should be justified in the medical records.*

Dying declarations

Under common law a dying declaration can be accepted in evidence provided the judge is satisfied that the deceased was aware of his/her being in a dying state at the time he made the declaration. That is, they believe that death is imminent. The declaration can be made to a police officer if they are present or to a HCP. Therefore the HCP should document any comments the patient makes to them (in the patient's own words) as at a later time this can be given in evidence in court.

Blood samples and the police

> **Case study 13.1 Pre-transfusion blood samples**
>
> A 40-year-old man is brought to the ED following a fight at a football match. He has sustained a stab wound to his face, a head injury and a number of wounds to his arms and hands. Following the primary assessment and resuscitation the patient is awaiting a CT scan. A police officer involved with the case arrives at the ED and asks the nurse caring for the patient for a pre-transfusion sample of his blood. The nurse is unsure if she should do this, and seeks advice from the nurse in charge.

In the ED it is not unusual for police officers to ask for a pre-transfusion blood sample to be taken or for samples taken for clinical care to be given to them. *Blood samples should not be handed to police officers without a court order from a judge,* unless the ED has pre-determined protocols and the HCP is familiar with them. The HCP must document the outcome of any such request.

The Police Reform Act 2002 changed the way blood samples for testing of alcohol and drugs are taken:

- A police constable makes the decision as to the competency of the patient to consent to the taking of a blood sample to test for alcohol and drugs. This is usually following a road traffic collision.
- The blood taken from an existing line is not acceptable and police have no powers to take and test blood that has been taken as part of the patient's care.
- The treating doctor is informed and can object if taking the blood would be prejudicial to care, and in trauma resuscitations this needs to be considered.
- Blood can be taken by a forensic medical examiner (FME) if a police constable has assessed the patient as incapable of giving consent (for medical reasons).

- The FME is satisfied that the person is not able to consent (for whatever reason).
- If an FME is not available then *a hospital doctor* can undertake the procedure (it cannot be delegated to another HCP) if he is not linked to the care or treatment of the patient.
- The doctor should document decisions if the patient is unable to consent and must be familiar with and use a special kit.
- This blood is then taken but not tested until the patient can consent.

Police family liaison officers

These are police officers who come from a variety of policing backgrounds, volunteer for the role and undertake specific training. They are primarily investigators and they are an important link between the investigating team and the family, providing support and information. They are usually deployed for:

- Suspected homicides
- Critical incidents
- Major incidents
- Road traffic collisions.

In some circumstances they are responsible for gathering information from the family to assist with identification. They may accompany family members to the hospital and remain with them during discussions with HCPs, and they may also accompany the family during the viewing of the deceased.

DISCLOSURE TO OTHER AGENCIES

The work of the ED exposes all ED staff to constant requests for information from various agencies either in person or by telephone. *No information should be given over the telephone or in person unless the HCP is satisfied that the person they are speaking to is entitled to the information and the HCP is sure that patient confidentiality is not being breached.*

ORGAN AND TISSUE DONATION

Considering organ donation in the context of ED work does not seem to sit easily and there are often misconceptions as to what role the ED has in identifying when there is potential for a donation. Because of the continuing shortages of organs and tissue for transplantation the Department of Health has issued a 10 year plan to maximise organ donation which includes looking at ways to recover organs from those who have died suddenly following a cardiac event or trauma.[12]

The Human Tissue Act 2004 made it lawful for certain steps to be taken to preserve organs until information about the deceased's wishes could be obtained and if necessary to obtain consent from a family member. The Act also gave precedence to the deceased's wishes over that of the family and if the deceased had registered with the organ donor register or carried a donor card then family consent is not required for removal of organs. However in most circumstances, where family object, their wishes are respected.

The traditional source of organs is from those who have been diagnosed with brainstem death in the intensive care unit where the potential for donation is recognised and the transplant coordinator is informed while the patient is being ventilated. These are called heart beating donors.

In some EDs, patients who are dead on arrival or die in the department can donate kidneys, tissue and cells. The kidneys are preserved by inserting a femoral cannula and perfusing the kidneys with a preservative fluid. This allows time for family to be contacted and the deceased's wishes to be established. These are called non heart beating donors.

A donor can donate their kidneys (one or both), heart, lungs (one or both), liver, pancreas and small bowel, as well as tissue including corneas, heart valves, bone, skin and connective tissue. However, time considerations apply when transplanting tissue and organs (Box 13.1)

There are only two conditions where organ donation is ruled out completely. A person cannot become an organ or tissue donor if they have human immunodeficiency virus

---

> **Box 13.1 Time considerations for organ and tissue donation**
>
> - Heart and lungs need to be transplanted within 4–5 hours of removal from the donor
> - Livers should be transplanted within 9–10 hours of removal from the donor
> - Kidneys should be transplanted within 24 hours of removal though this can be extended up to 48 hours
>
> Some tissue can be stored for greater lengths of time but must be removed within certain time limits:
>
> - Corneas should ideally be removed within 12 hours, but it is possible to do so up to 24 hours
> - Heart valves should be removed within 48 hours so long as the body is refrigerated within 6 hours
> - Bone, skin, tendon and cartilage should be removed within 24 hours, again as long as the body is refrigerated within 6 hours

(HIV) or have, or are suspected of having, Creutzfeldt–Jakob disease (CJD). There is no minimum age to joining the NHS Organ Donor Register. Parents and guardians can register their children and children can register themselves. Children who are under 12 in Scotland and under 18 in the rest of the UK at the time of registration will require their parents' or guardians' agreement for donation to take place[13]

In the ED a family member may indicate to a HCP that the patient wished to donate organs, carried a donor card or had registered as a donor. It would be appropriate for the consultant in charge of care to be informed and contact made with the local transplant coordinator. The transplant coordinator can then give advice and guidance and may attend the ED. They will liaise with UK Transplant regarding would-be recipients. Donor death has to be certified by two senior doctors.

The coroner must be consulted before any decisions regarding organ donation are made. The coroner has to be satisfied that the removal of organs or tissue will not interfere with the investigation of the death (identification, cause of death and circumstances and includes criminal investigations).

Families may inform the HCP that their relative has agreed to leave their body 'to medical science' or their brain to a brain bank (usually those who suffered from Alzheimer's disease or Parkinson's disease). Again, it is very important that the coroner is informed of this early.

FORENSIC EVIDENCE

Preserving forensic evidence has never featured in the care of the trauma patient although clothing and sometimes blood samples have been handed to police officers with little thought to why this is done and the consequent legal implications. Anything and everything that can help to establish facts relating to any situation including a crime can be produced as evidence in a court. Preserving evidence is not only about convicting the guilty but also clearing the innocent and also establishing the circumstances, identification and cause of death of the deceased.

Resuscitation and life saving procedures must take precedence over the preservation of evidence but consideration should be given to reduce the loss of evidence.

Evidence abounds on, in and around the trauma patient attending the ED and this evidence can be lost, changed or destroyed during the process of resuscitation and care. The police investigate crime and may rely on evidence from the ED to assist in this process. However, they need to be able to show a chain of custody (continuity) and proof that no alteration of the inherent quality or composition of the evidence has occurred.

The coroner has a duty to hold an inquest if he has a body lying in his district and there is reasonable cause to suspect that the death was violent or unnatural[14] and the coroner will be reliant on evidence from the ED to establish the facts surrounding this death, the medical cause of death and the identity of the deceased.

Evidence can fall into a number of categories:

- Visual
- Physical
- Trace
- Biological
- Behavioural.

Visual

This is anything that is visible that the HCP can see on, in or around the body. It may be marks, injuries or signs, which fade and heal with time resulting in lost evidence if the patient survives and subsequently dies later. Remember that some cases come to court years after the incident when no bruises, scratches, injuries or marks remain, therefore accurate recording at the time will assist the HCP and the courts to establish circumstances. Most EDs follow established protocols in managing the trauma patient[15] and the completion of the secondary survey would assist in trapping the minor injuries and marks that are often overlooked. Consideration needs to be given as to the best means to record this visual evidence and a lot will be gained from well written notes, drawings and/or photographs:

- If written, the mark should be described accurately in terms of appearance, colour, size, location (in relation to anatomical site), shape and edge characteristics. This is relatively simple if there are few, uncomplicated marks but difficulties may arise when there are multiple marks with varying characteristics.
- Drawing diagrams demands some accuracy but may complement the written word and give a more accurate description.
- The gold standard would be to take a photograph, with a measurable object (coin, ruler) included. With digital photography the photograph can be incorporated into electronic and paper records and continuity is ensured as no film needs to be developed. However, consideration

needs to be given to issues of consent and confidentiality and therefore ED departments should have a written policy that would cover the taking of clinical and evidential photographs.[16,17]

- Any wound should be covered with a clean dry dressing without washing or cleaning the area.

Recording these marks supposes correct use of medical terminology and this doesn't always come easy to HCPs.[18–21] The circumstances of the injury are not always evident to ED staff so there should be no assumptions:

- *Laceration: Caused by blunt trauma* which tears, shears and crushes tissue and the edges are irregular with bleeding infiltration. Tissue bridges and debris imbedded in the injury are also characteristic.
- *Incision: Caused by sharp objects*, cuts and divides, edges are clean and there is usually no bleeding infiltration. The use of the terms penetrating injuries or stab injury is correct under incision, the difference being a penetrating or stab injury is usually deeper than it is wide.
- *Bruise: Caused by blunt trauma*, a subcutaneous collection of blood which may show the pattern of the inflicting implement.
- *Abrasion (grazes, scratches):* A superficial injury to the epidermis which may be from grinding or sliding. For example when a person 'grazes' their knee in a fall, the direction of the fall can be noted. An abrasion may also show an imprint of an object or the surface making contact at the time of the injury.
- *Bites:* Can vary from clear tooth marks to insignificant bruises.
- *Burns:* Can vary from minor skin redness to full thickness of the skin. May show patterning or distinctive marks of objects used, e.g. cigarette burns.
- *Any old healing wounds:* Abrasions, bites and burns should also be noted as these may have significance in, for example, suspected non-accidental injuries (both adult and children).

- *Sexual assault wounds:* May vary from visible vaginal, anal, penile injuries to internal injuries to bite marks on breasts or other parts of the body, or a patient informing the HCP that they have been raped. The HCP should not make assumptions and refer their observations to senior staff. Wounds present should be described as above and what the patient says should be documented in the patient's own words. The HCP can assist in evidence preservation by placing clean dry dressings over the wounds without cleaning or washing the area.
- *Firearm wounds:* Can be caused by:
  - Smooth bore weapons (shotguns – where bullets contain shot pellets) or
  - Rifled weapons (pistols, revolvers and rifles where the bullets are solid)

  The characteristics of the wounds these weapons cause vary enormously and depend on the distance from the weapon when fired, type and velocity of the bullet. There may be only one wound or any number of entry and exit wounds, or widespread disruption. The HCP is advised to describe the injuries, call them wounds and leave the actual classification of entry/exit, type of weapon and bullet to the ballistic expert and the forensic pathologist.

The term wound has been legally defined and could be described as 'an injury involving a full thickness breach of the skin'.[18] This term *could be used to describe any laceration, incision or a gunshot injury where the HCP is uncertain of the correct terminology or the circumstances in which the injury was sustained.*

Physical

These are the visible 'bits and pieces' that accompany the patient into the ED and can be in, on, around the body and clothes. This may be bits of glass, car pieces, pellets, bullets (or part of), debris, shrapnel, perhaps a weapon, personal documents and personal effects. This evidence is easily lost, particularly in the clean up process after the patient has moved on, and can be easily contaminated with other ED debris and incorrect handling.

In order to preserve this type of evidence the HCP should consider:

- Minimal handling of the object
- Place in a clean bag, box or specimen jar
- Label the container – where and when found and by whom. Describe the object, sign and seal it
- Record on a property document
- Record in the medical records including where it can be found
- If a police officer requests the object – consider if consent is required, and then, if given to the police, record in the medical records the name of the police officer, their rank and if in uniform their shoulder number and the time/date. The police officer should sign that he has taken it. This ensures the chain of custody.

Clothing

The clothing the patient is or was wearing contains a multitude of evidence (including visual, physical, trace, biological) that will be irretrievably lost, change or destroyed by poor handling. The defects, tears and rips, missing buttons, soot, debris and blood splatters all provide a piece in the jigsaw of establishing the circumstances and includes contents of pockets which may also assist in establishing identity. Clothing also includes cycle and motorcycle helmets, glasses, sunglasses and shoes. The clothing worn by road users assists in establishing identification, visibility on the road at the time of the incident and marks of contact with other objects or vehicles. The clothing and footwear worn in the exercise of an employment may have implications for the employer if it was inappropriate, incorrectly worn or not present at all.

Cutting off the clothes in an emergency is acceptable but how this is done and what happens to the clothing afterwards will determine whether evidence has been preserved:

- Avoid cutting through any defects (holes).
- Avoid cutting through any blood spatters or patterns.
- Document that the clothing has been cut off (so there is no confusion as to the provenance of the cut and that it is not taken to be a cut or tear occurring in the course of a struggle).
- *Do not drop the clothes on the floor* – the floor is covered in minute debris of the day's emergencies and contaminates the clothing.
- Fold minimally.
- Put into clean bag, preferably paper or evidence bags available from the police or on to a clean surface until emergency is over. The police would prefer that each item of clothing goes into a separate bag.
- Check and document all items on a property form or in the medical notes with a colleague and sign the form.
- *If the police request the clothing then ensure that the police officer signs the property form and includes his rank and if in uniform his shoulder number.*
- *Otherwise the clothing should accompany the body to the mortuary or should be made available to the coroner.*

Trace evidence

This is the minute, barely visible evidence that includes fibres, loose hair, soot, paint chips, glass, blood splatters and saliva which may relate to the place from where the patient came or another with whom contact had been made. It is easily contaminated and lost and is very difficult to protect and preserve in the ED in a trauma resuscitation, however the HCP can take steps to reduce the contamination and loss of this type of evidence by:

- Taking care of the clothing as above.
- Taking and retaining the sheets, blankets and the body bag as above.
- The police may request that bags are put onto the hands and sealed. This protects evidence which may include soot

---

Box 13.2 DNA and elimination of substances from the body

- DNA is affected if any blood is given and includes O negative, type specific and matched
- Alcohol is diluted and metabolised 15 mg/100 ml/hr
- Carbon monoxide is eliminated in 40 mins if oxygen is given at 100%

---

if a firearm has been discharged, or debris, blood and tissue under the nails or broken nails and small defence injuries.
- Covering any wounds with clean dry dressings without cleaning or washing the area.

Biological

This is any bodily fluid or substance which can be analysed to establish blood groups, DNA, and/or the presence of poisons, solvents, gases, alcohol and drugs (prescribed, illicit, other). In the ED this would essentially be blood and urine that can be lost, contaminated or change (Box 13.2).

When taking a sample it should be:

- Pre-transfusion
- Pre-dilution
- Pre-metabolism
- Pre-elimination.

The blood samples taken on admission *may* be used to establish evidence of a crime and also to establish the cause or circumstances of the death, therefore when taking blood or urine samples the following steps should be adhered to:

- Correctly label the container with patient's name, hospital number, date and time that the sample is taken and the name of the HCP taking the sample.
- Document the means of transport to the laboratory for continuity purposes.

- Inform the laboratory that the sample may be required for medicolegal purposes.
- Following a death the blood can be released to the coroner following established protocols with the hospital laboratories.
- The police do not have the right of taking this blood unless they have established protocols with the hospital laboratory and/or they have a court order authorising the release of the blood for investigation purposes.

Establishing that the blood sample is pre-transfusion supposes that that the first blood sample taken on the arrival in the ED was intended to establish the blood group, blood characteristics and chemistry to guide treatment. *Documentation that the blood was indeed taken before any blood products were administered would assist in preserving this evidence.*

Behavioural
In a trauma resuscitation it may not be possible to remark on demeanour or attitude, however the patient may say something that seems unusual or there may be unusual odours. The HCP should document anything that they find unusual using the patient's or the accompanying person's own words. HCPs must not make assumptions and should avoid the use of the term 'alleges'.

In some cases hearsay evidence, 'any statement not made in oral evidence in the proceedings,'[22] may be admissible in a coroner's court and also in other courts although the decision will rest with the presiding judge.[23]

DOCUMENTATION
All trauma documentation should be comprehensive, comprehensible and a permanent record of what has happened to the patient along the continuum of care. If the trauma case is to go to court then this will usually take months, if not years. Therefore what is written will provide the facts and perhaps

the HCP's defence for the future, as memory cannot be relied on.

Whatever happens during a trauma resuscitation it is imperative that all actions are recorded. In emergencies it is accepted that recording will not be contemporaneous but must occur as soon as reasonably possible. If records are poor and lacking in detail then establishing what care was given, or not, is impossible and, essentially, the HCP would be in difficulty in defending their actions or decisions. If their conduct or care is in question then it would be very difficult for a lawyer to defend if scant notes are made. The maxim 'if it isn't written down then it wasn't done' is still used to challenge the actions of HCPs.

There is only one original medical record and therefore courts all work with photocopies (copies for the lawyers, the judge, coroner, expert witnesses, jury for example). Therefore the HCP should:

- Make no assumptions.
- Remain objective.
- Avoid abbreviations as although HCPs may understand what is meant the lawyers, jury, judge, coroner, family may not. Abbreviations may save time but they can be interpreted differently by different people, and therefore making sense of the record is time consuming and could compromise communication and care.[24]
- Use dark coloured pens and write legibly.
- Keep all writing within the margins of the A4 size paper. Writing laboratory results, and any other documentation, in margins and at the very top and bottom of pages risks the loss of information in the copying procedure and merely serves to frustrate the courts in their search for the truth. Also interpretation of trends, treatment decisions and laboratory results is rendered difficult.
- Record times including the time the patient actually *arrived* in the ED, when seen by clinicians, times to and from other departments.

- Record all medical interventions and their position, e.g. chest drains, central lines.
- Record samples, clothing and any 'evidence' taken, what has happened to them and where they can be found. Include a signature of the receiver if handed to the coroner's officer or police officer.
- Record decision making process if a prescribed treatment is not done.
- Ensure observation charts, fluid and drug charts are included – these will also be copied, scrutinised and analysed to identify trends.
- All printouts from electronic machines and the electronic records should be included in the medical records.
- Any photographs taken should be attached and include time taken and by whom.
- If police ask to speak to the patient, record the decision and if access is denied, then document why.
- HCPs must always sign their record and print their name legibly.

If the HCP is requested to write a report or make a statement for the police, a solicitor or the coroner, then they should establish if they are the right person to do it and that it is clear what is required.

Then ensure that the report is:

- Accurate and based on the HCP's record entries
- Legible and free of ambiguous jargon and abbreviations
- Comprehensible
- Objective and devoid of opinion
- The hospital trust's legal department and the ED manager are satisfied with what is written
- *The HCP should be prepared to go to court.*

CARE OF THE RELATIVES
This is a challenging aspect of trauma care, whether the patient has survived the initial injury or not, and there are many important factors to consider:

- HCPs should remember that all communications, seemingly insensitive remarks and perceptions of care given are usually remembered by relatives for years after the traumatic event. Therefore the HCP should remain compassionate, sensitive and understanding throughout their interaction with family in the ED.
- The use of an appropriate interpreter or advocate is indicated if English is not the first language of the family.
- The term 'relatives' or 'family' is used in the broadest sense and may include very close friends, extended family, informal partnerships or the legal civil partnership.[25]
- Care and support of bereaved people has not always been well managed,[26–28] however guidance has been developed which sets out the principles underpinning the provision of services and professional practice around the time of death and afterwards.[29]
- A trauma death is always sudden and unexpected and differs from an expected death in that the families have not had time to prepare for the event.[30]
- Bereaved peoples' grief reactions vary considerably. How they will react is difficult to predict and their emotional vulnerability must be managed in such a way as to not cause further distress.
- Bereaved people sometimes have difficulty in remembering information so the HCP should consider writing information down or giving the bereaved person some paper and a pen to take notes.
- Difficulties may arise for HCPs in the ED in establishing the legitimacy of a relationship and caution should be exercised in the early stages until the relationship is clarified.
- Who tells the relative (of the death, outcome of care or prognosis) and how they are told will depend on the circumstances but when the family are in the ED they require a quiet room and information should be given by the most appropriate person in the ED. This could be the trauma team leader, the lead consultant or a designated person.[31]

- Consideration also needs to be given as to how a family member and the deceased is addressed. This should be established very early and this name used rather than referring to the person as 'the body', 'the deceased', or the 'patient'.
- Children should not be excluded from these discussions or from seeing the dead person if they wish.[30,32]
- Information must be honest, accurate and transparent using terminology that is unambiguous, e.g. 'He has died' rather than 'we lost him'.
- If a mistake has been made, experience at coroners' inquests suggests that families invariably want an explanation, an apology, compensation and that 'it should not happen to others'.[33,34]
- In some societies death is not the end but a transition to another state and is usually accompanied by some ritual to assist the transition period and the mourning and grieving process.[35,36] Society is multicultural, multireligious and interwoven with community and personal beliefs. How a trauma-related death is managed in the ED will have an impact on the family and the community, so some thought needs to be given to what rituals can or cannot be allowed.
- The family's requirements should be discussed with the coroner/coroner's officer who will assist the HCP in determining what is acceptable. Any decision should be explained to the family.
- Most people would want to see their dead relative and how this is managed depends on the circumstances. Protocols need to be established with the coroner as to how and when this should occur. It can occur in the ED, in the hospital mortuary and it may well be the responsibility of a member of the ED staff to accompany the family. In some circumstances a police officer or a coroner's officer may attend with the family.
- The HCP should be wary of giving information to families on coroner's procedures as this may conflict with the coroner's decision and cause distress to families. For example

although the death is being reported to the coroner it does not necessarily follow that a post mortem will occur.

- It would be helpful if the family member was given *in writing* the contact name and telephone number for the coroners' office.
- If police family liaison officers are present then they may remain with the family throughout any discussions.

CONCLUSION

ED staff have a duty to save life and cause no further harm and therefore focusing on saving a life takes priority over any requirements of the other agencies involved. The HCP involved in trauma care should be familiar with issues of consent, confidentiality and disclosure and the requirements of the agencies involved in death procedures. They should also be able to support, care for and inform bereaved people of what has happened and what may happen following a death.

Understanding the coroner and police requirements, protecting and preserving the evidence and considering organ and tissue donation are all-important aspects of trauma care. Inquiries into trauma deaths contribute to the understanding of injury patterns, treatment outcomes and injury prevention, therefore the HCP should assist in gathering information for this process.

Establishing protocols that are acceptable to the ED, the legal department, the healthcare trust, the coroner and the police should make the process an integral facet of trauma care. It should also make managing a trauma-related death less stressful for the HCP.

KEY INFORMATION BOX

- All trauma-related deaths should be reported to the coroner irrespective of where or when the injury leading to the death occurred
- Resuscitation and life saving procedures must take precedence over the preservation of evidence but

consideration needs to be given as to how to minimise the loss, change or contamination of evidence
- No clothing or property should be given to next of kin or family unless it is established that neither the police nor the coroner require it
- Use correct terminology when describing injuries and wounds
- Ensure all documentation is comprehensive, comprehensible and permanent
- Blood samples cannot be handed to police officers without a court order from a judge *unless* specific protocols are in place.

REFERENCES

1. Health and Safety Commission (2007) Statistics of fatal injuries 2006/7. National Statistics
2. Nicholas S, Kershaw C, Walker A (2007) Crime in England and Wales 2006. Home Office Statistical Bulletin 11/07 (2nd edn)
3. Department of Transport (2006) Transport Statistics Bulletin (07) 18. Road Casualties in Great Britain Main Results 2006. National Statistics
4. Allen R (2007) Department of Constitutional Affairs statistics on deaths reported to coroners in England and Wales 2006. DCA Statistical Bulletin
5. Coroners Act 1988 s 8(1), Coroners rules 1984
6. Dorries C (2004) Coroners courts: a guide to law and practice. (2nd edn). Oxford University Press, Oxford
7. Department of Health (1998) Chief Medical Officers Update 20. Department of Health, London
8. Department of Health (2003) 33837/National Health Service Code of Practice: confidentiality. Department of Health, London
9. Department of Health (2006) 277311 The Caldicott Guardian Manual. UK Council of Caldicott Guardians, London
10. British Medical Association (1999) Disclosure in the public interest. http://www.bma.org.uk/ap.nsf/Content/Confidentialtydisclosure

11. General Medical Council (2003) Reporting of gunshot wounds guidance for doctors in emergency departments. http://www.gmc-uk.org/guidance/current/library/reporting_gunshot_wounds.asp

12. Department of Health (2003) Saving lives, valuing donors – a transplant framework for England. Department of Health, London

13. UK Transplant, Communications Directorate, Fox Den Road, Stoke Gifford, Bristol BS34 8RR

14. Section 8(i)(a) Coroners Act 1984

15. American College of Surgeons (2004) Initial assessment and management. In: Advanced trauma life support for doctors. Student course manual (7th edn), 11–32. American College of Surgeons, Chicago

16. Bhangoo P, Maconochie I, Batrick N, Henry E (2005) Taking pictures – a survey of current practice in emergency departments and proposed recommendations for best practice. Emergency Medical Journal 22:761–765

17. General Medical Council (2002) Making and using visual and audio recordings of patients. http://www.gmc-uk.org/guidance/current/library/making_audiovisual.asp

18. Capper C (2001) The language of forensic medicine: the meaning of some terms employed. Medicine, Science and the Law 41:256–259

19. Rutty G (2000) Interpretation of wounds. Nursing Times 96(31):41–42

20. Machin V, Levington F, Dean P (2003) Preparing a police statement. In: Medico legal pocket book, 27–37. Churchill Livingstone/Elsevier Science, Oxford

21. Jones R (2003) Wound and injury awareness amongst students and doctors. Journal of Clinical Forensic Medicine 10:231–234

22. The Criminal Justice Act 2003 section 114

23. The Criminal Justice Act 2003 section 116

24. Davies NM (2005) Medical abbreviations: 26,000 conveniences at the expense of communications and safety (12th edn). Neil M Davies Associates, Pennsylvania

25. Civil Partnership Act 2004
26. Department of Health (2001) The report of the public enquiry into childrens heart surgery at Bristol Royal Infirmary 1984–1995. Department of Health, London
27. Department of Health (2001) The Royal Liverpool Childrens Enquiry Report. Department of Health, London
28. Royal College of Pathologists and Royal College of Paediatrics and Child Health (2004) Sudden unexpected death in infancy. A multi-agency protocol for care and investigation. http://www.rcpath.org/index.asp
29. Department of Health (2005) When a patient dies. Advice on developing bereavement services in the NHS. Department of Health, London
30. Faulkner A (2003) Working with bereaved people. Churchill Livingston/Elsevier Science, Oxford
31. Dabrowski G, Anderson H (2002) Legal, ethical and family issues. In: The trauma manual (2nd edn) (Eds Peitzman AB, Rhodes M, Schwab CW, Yealy DM, Fabian TC), 508–512. Lippincott, Williams & Wilkins, Philadelphia
32. Young B, Papadatou D (1997) Childhood death and bereavement across cultures, In: Murray Parkes C, Laungani P, Young B (eds) Death and bereavement across cultures, 191–205. Routledge, London
33. Davis G, Lindsey R, Seabourne G, Griffiths-Baker J (2002) Experiencing Inquests, Home Office Research Study 241. Home Office Research, Development and Statistics Department, London
34. Hill R, Crouch J (2006) IPSOS MORI, users experiences of coroners courts. DCA research series 6/06. Department for Constitutional Affairs, London
35. Rosenblatt P (1997) Grief in small-scale societies. In: Death and bereavement across cultures (Eds Murray Parkes C, Laungani P, Young B), 27–51. Routledge, London
36. Murray Parkes C (1997) Help for the dying and the bereaved. In: Death and bereavement across cultures (Eds Murray Parkes C, Laungani P, Young B), 206–217. Routledge, London

Index